All About Herbs, Charcoal, Medications, and Drugs

I0407136

a

Spirit of Prophecy Compilation

(Now with Improved Text and Indices)

by

Vernon Sparks, M.D.

Copyright © 1999, 2002, 2007, 2011

by
Vernon Sparks

Published
by

Digital Inspiration
1481 Reagan Valley Road
Tellico Plains, TN 37385

www.vsdigitalinspiration.com

Contents

Introduction

IN the writings of the Spirit of Prophecy there are found repeated condemnations of the use of tea and coffee as beverages. Yet, Ellen White states that on rare occasions she resorted to the use of tea or coffee as a medicine. Her writings also roundly condemn the use of "drugs," especially of "poisonous" drugs. Yet, she is quoted as stating that "if quinine will save life, use quinine." See Appendix B.

This present volume is a comprehensive compilation of the Spirit of Prophecy counsels regarding drugs, medications, herbs, stimulants, narcotics, charcoal, and related subjects. A knowledge of God's will can only be arrived at on this subject, just as with any doctrinal teaching, by a study of, and a harmonization of, all of the available counsel. Even with such a study, the seeker of truth, will need the continued guidance of the Holy Spirit to know how to apply these counsels to the varying circumstances of daily life.

Willie White, the son of the prophetess, points out the importance of taking into account the circumstances surrounding the giving of the inspired directions:

"One of the most perplexing problems we have to deal with in preparing Mother's writings for publication is in just such matters as this, where the conditions of a family, or a church, or an institution are presented to her, and warnings and instruction are given regarding these conditions. In such cases, Mother writes clearly and forcefully, and without qualification regarding the situation presented to her. And it is a great blessing to us to have this instruction for our study in dealing with similar conditions elsewhere.

"But when we take what she has written, and publish it without any description, or particular reference to the conditions existing when and where the testimony was given, there is always the possibility of the instruction being used as applying {385} to places and conditions that are very different.

"Very much perplexity has been brought into our work in this way, by the use of what Mother has written on the subject of diet, and on the use of drugs, and on other subjects that you will think of without my enumerating them; and when the time has come for instruction to be given to some individual, or family, or church, which presented the right course to be taken, under conditions which were different from those contemplated in former writings, the exception made, or the different course advised in view of the different conditions, has often come as a surprise to those who felt that the instruction they have been studying was of universal application." *The Ellen G. White Biography,* 1905–1915, vol. 6, 384–385.

The reader of this book will probably indeed be "surprised" by some of the information presented. To understand the medical practices of Ellen White's day the reader is directed to Appendix H, "Treating Fire With Fire," and pages 13–27 of the book *The Story of Our Health Message* by Doris Robinson. Also, a chapter from an Adventist home, health care book entitled *Home and Health—A Household Manual,* published by the Pacific Press Publishing House in 1907, is reproduced in Appendix F. The reader will find the counsel of that volume to be much out of harmony with that in Appendix G which is from a non-Adventist home health care publication of the same era.

The compiler of this present book is in the possession of a 1500-page, 2 volume, publication entitled *Health Knowledge.* This set was printed in 1927. Selected pages from this work are reproduced in Appendix G. Many will be surprised to find that indeed, "poisonous drugs" such as arsenic, mercury, morphine, quinine, opium, strychnine, and even potassium cyanide were, at that late date, still commonly being used.

We need to be aware that Ellen White lived and wrote in an era when many of the over-the-counter, patent medicines and the alcoholic drinks contained very addictive drugs such as opium, morphine, and so on. Even the "soft drink" Coca Cola contained cocaine in its original formulation.

An attempt has been made to list the counsels in chronological order. The date preceding each reference is when the incident occurred or the counsel was first published. This publication does not include all of the inspired counsels regarding tobacco, tea, or coffee, but only those paragraphs that identify them as drugs, narcotics, stimulants, and so forth. Neither does this book include all instruction regarding the natural remedies such as pure air, water, etc. unless they are specified as being medicine or medication. All capitalization of key words is for emphasis by the present compiler. The numbers in curly brackets such as {131} indicate where a new page begins in the original sources.

It is the prayer of the compiler that this book will be of benefit to each reader to more fully understand God's will regarding this important subject.

Vernon Sparks

Spirit of Prophecy References

"And by the river upon the bank thereof, on this side and on that side, shall grow all trees for meat, whose leaf shall not fade, neither shall the fruit thereof be consumed: it shall bring forth new fruit according to his months, because their waters they issued out of the sanctuary: and the fruit thereof shall be for meat, and the leaf thereof for MEDICINE." Ezekiel 47:12.

1851—*The Ellen G. White Biography*, 1827–1862, vol. 1, 224.

"I have seen in vision that TOBACCO was a filthy weed, and that it must be laid aside or given up. Said my accompanying angel, 'If it is an idol, it is high time it was given up, and unless it is given up, the frown of God will be upon the one that uses it, and he cannot be sealed with the seal of the living God. If it is used as a MEDICINE, go to God; He is the Great Physician, and those that use the FILTHY WEED for MEDICINE greatly dishonor God. 'There is a balm in Gilead, there is a Physician there. Be ye clean that bear the vessels of the Lord.' "
(*Manuscript Releases*, vol. 5, 377).

1854—*Testimonies*, vol. 1, 92–94.

"About this time a celebrated physician who gave counsel free visited Rochester, and I decided to have him examine my eye. He thought the swelling would prove to be a cancer. But upon feeling my pulse, he said: 'You are much diseased, and will die of apoplexy before that swelling shall break out. You are in a dangerous condition with disease of the heart.' This did not startle me, for I had been aware that without speedy relief I must go down to the grave. Two other women who had come for counsel were suffering with the same disease. The physician said that I was in a more dangerous condition than either of them, and it could not be more than three weeks before I would be afflicted with paralysis. I asked if he thought his MEDICINE would cure me. He did not give me much encouragement. I tried the remedies which he prescribed, but received no benefit. . . . {94}
(*Life Sketches of James White and Ellen G. White (1880 edition)*, 305.)

"Again I visited the physician, and as soon as he felt my pulse, he

said: 'Madam, an entire change has taken place in your system; but the two women who visited me for counsel when you were last here are dead.' I stated to him that his MEDICINE had not cured me, as I could take none of it. After I left, the doctor said to a friend of mine: 'Her case is a mystery. I do not understand it.' "
(*Life Sketches of James White and Ellen G. White (1880 edition)*, 307)

1854—*Spiritual Gifts*, vol. 2, 185, 187–188.

"A celebrated physician visited Rochester who gave counsel free. I decided to have him examine my eye. He thought the swelling would prove to be a cancer. He felt my pulse, and said, 'You are much diseased, and will die of apoplexy before that swelling will break out. You are in a dangerous condition with disease of the heart.' This did not startle me, for I had been aware that unless I received speedy relief I must lie in the grave. Two other females had come for counsel who were suffering with the same disease. The physician said that I was in a more dangerous condition than either of them, and it could not be more than three weeks before I would be afflicted with paralysis, and next would follow apoplexy. I inquired if he thought his MEDICINE would cure me. He did not give me much encouragement. I purchased some of his MEDICINE. The eyewash was very painful, and I received no benefit from it. I was unable to use the remedies the physician prescribed. . . . {187}

"Again I visited the physician, and as soon as he felt my pulse he said, 'Madam, you are better. An entire change has taken place in your system; but the two women who visited me for counsel when you were last here are dead.' I told him it was not his MEDICINE that {188} had cured me, for I could use none of it. And as I was about to relate the wonderful dealings of the Lord with me, a poor laborer rushed into the room, almost beside himself, saying, 'Doctor, they say I must die! that I am in consumption!' Large drops of sweat stood upon his brow. The physician tried to calm his excited mind while he examined his lungs. He waited his examination with intense anxiety. The physician shook his head, and told him he could not deceive him; that he had the quick consumption, and must soon die. His feelings overcame him, and he burst into tears. He had no hope in God, and the future to him was a fearful uncertainty. I was obliged to leave. Sister P., who now rests in the grave, had accompanied me, and related to the physician after I left, that the Lord had heard prayer for me, and restored me to health. Said he, 'Her case is a mystery. I do not understand it.' "

1856—*Spiritual Gifts*, vol. 2, 202.

"We have felt the power and blessing of God for a few weeks past. God has been very merciful. He has wrought in a wonderful manner for my husband. We have brought him to our Great Physician in the arms of our faith, and like blind Bartimaeus have cried. 'Jesus, thou son of David, have mercy on me' (Mark 10:47); and we have been comforted. The healing power of God has been felt. ALL MEDICINE has been laid aside, and we rely alone upon the arm of our Great Physician. We are not yet satisfied. Our faith says, Entire restoration. We have seen the salvation of God, yet we expect to see and feel more. I believe without a doubt that my husband will yet be able to sound the last notes of warning to the world. For weeks past our peace has been like a river. Our souls triumph in God. Gratitude, unspeakable gratitude fills my soul for the tokens of God's love which we have of late felt and seen. We feel like dedicating ourselves anew to God."

(Life Sketches of James White and Ellen G. White (1880 edition), 317; Review and Herald, January 10, 1856)

1856—*The Ellen G. White Biography*, 1827–1862, vol. 1, 335–336.

"God has wrought for us in a remarkable manner since the conference. My husband has been much afflicted. Incessant labor has nearly carried him to the grave. But our prayers have ascended to God morning, noon, and night for his restoration. ALL MEDICINE has been entirely laid aside, and we have brought him in the arms of our faith to our skillful Physician. We have been heard and answered. An entire change has been wrought {336} for him. . . . We believe without a doubt, if he is careful of the health God has given him, his strength will increase and he will be able to overcome the disease that has fastened upon him."

1860—*Spiritual Gifts*, vol. 2, 104–106.

"At Middletown we met sister Bonfoey and our little Henry. My child grew feeble. We had used SIMPLE HERBS, but they had no effect. The neighbors who came in said we could not {105} keep him long, for he would die with consumption. One advised us to use one MEDICINE, another something else. But it did not effect the child favorably. Finally he could take no nourishment. Townsend's SARSAPARILLA was recommended as the last resort. We concluded to try it. We could send by a friend to Hartford that day, and must decide in a few moments. I went before the Lord in my room alone, and while praying obtained the evidence that our only Source of help was in the Lord. If he did not bless,

and heal the child, MEDICINE could not save him.
(*Life Sketches of James White and Ellen G. White (1880 edition)*, 253.)

"I there decided to venture the life of the child upon the promises of God. I had a lively sense of his willingness and power to save, and there alone before God cried out, 'We will believe, and show to these unbelieving neighbors, who are expecting the death of the child, that there is a God in Israel, whose ear is open to the prayers of his children. We will trust alone in thee.' I felt the power of God to that degree that for a short time I was helpless. My husband opened the door to say to me that the friend was waiting for our decision. 'Shall we get the SARSAPARILLA?' I answered, 'No. Tell him we will try the strength of God's promises.'
(*Life Sketches of James White and Ellen G. White (1880 edition)*, 253.)

"The neighbors looked upon me with astonishment. They were confident the child would die. That night we anointed him, and my {106} husband prayed for him, laying his hands upon him in the name of the Lord. He looked up with a smile. A light seemed to rest upon his features, and we there had the evidence that the Lord had answered our prayers. We gave him no more MEDICINE. He gained strength fast, and the next day could stand upon his feet."
(*Life Sketches of James White and Ellen G. White (1880 edition)*, 254)

1860—*Spiritual Gifts*, vol. 2, 126–127.

"Not long after this, terrible fear seized this woman. A horror rested upon her, and she began to confess. She even went from house to house among her unbelieving neighbors, and confessed that the man she had been living with for years was not her husband, that she ran away from England and left a kind husband and one child. She also confessed that she had professed to understand MEDICINE, and had taken oath that the bottles of mixture she made cost her one dollar, when they cost her only twelve cents. Said that she had taken thirty dollars from a poor man by taking a false oath, and many such wicked acts she confessed, and her repentance seemed to be genuine. In {127} some cases she restored where she had taken away wrongfully. In one instance she started on foot forty miles to confess. We could see the hand of God in this matter. He gave her no rest day nor night, until she confessed her sins publicly, that God's work might be vindicated."

1862—*Testimonies*, vol. 1, 306–307.

"The husband should manifest great interest in his family. Especially should he be very tender of the feelings of a feeble wife. He can shut

the door against much disease. Kind, cheerful, and encouraging words will prove more effective than the most healing MEDICINES. These will bring courage to the heart of the desponding and discouraged, and the happiness and sunshine brought into the family by kind {307} acts and encouraging words will repay the effort tenfold. The husband should remember that much of the burden of training his children rests upon the mother, that she has much to do with molding their minds. This should call into exercise his tenderest feelings, and with care should he lighten her burdens. He should encourage her to lean upon his large affections, and direct her mind to Heaven, where there is strength and peace, and a final rest for the weary. He should not come to his home with a clouded brow, but should with his presence bring sunlight into the family, and should encourage his wife to look up and believe in God. Unitedly they can claim the promises of God and bring His rich blessing into the family. Unkindness, complaining, and anger shut Jesus from the dwelling. I saw that angels of God will flee from a house where there are unpleasant words, fretfulness, and strife."
(*Review and Herald*, April 22, 1862.
FP—*The Adventist Home*, 217–218; *Mind, Character, and Personality*, vol.1, 158.
MP—*My Life Today*, 152)

1863—*The Ellen G. White Biography*, 1862–1876, vol. 2, 16.

"Had we allowed ourselves to be smothered in close sleeping rooms, and given up to every pain and ache of the lungs, and throat, and head, and kept up a perpetual dosing with this and that MEDICINE, we might now be silent in death, or dragging out a miserable existence, of no benefit to anyone. Air, water, and light are God's great remedies. If the people would learn to use these, doctors and their DRUGS would be in less demand."

1863—*Selected Messages*, book 3, 280.

"I saw that it was a sacred duty to attend to our health, and arouse others to their duty, and yet not take the burden of their case upon us. Yet we have a duty to speak, to come out against intemperance of every kind—intemperance in working, in eating, in drinking, and in DRUGGING—and then point them to God's great MEDICINE, water, pure soft water, for diseases, for health, for cleanliness, and for a luxury."
(*Manuscript Releases*, vol. 5, 105; *The Ellen G. White Biography*, 1862–1876, vol. 2, 73)

1864—*A Solemn Appeal*, 62–63.

"The state of our world is alarming. Everywhere we look, we see imbecility, dwarfed {63} forms, crippled limbs, misshapen heads, and deformity of every description. Sin and crime, and the violation of nature's laws, are the causes of this accumulation of human woe and suffering. A large share of the youth now living are worthless. Corrupt habits are wasting their energies, and bringing upon them loathsome and complicated diseases. Unsuspecting parents will try the skill of physicians, one after another, who prescribe DRUGS, when they generally know the real cause of the failing health; but for fear of offending, and losing their fees, they keep silent, when, as faithful physicians, they should expose the real cause. Their DRUGS only add a second great burden for abused nature to struggle against; and in this struggle nature often breaks down in her efforts, and the victim dies. And the friends look upon the death as a mysterious dispensation of Providence, when the most mysterious part of the matter is, that nature bore up as long as she did against her violated laws. Health, reason, and life, were sacrificed to depraved lusts."

1864—*Spiritual Gifts*, vol. 4A, 130–131, 133–141, 145–146.

"Persons who have indulged their appetite to eat freely of meat, highly-seasoned gravies, and various kinds of rich cakes and preserves, cannot immediately relish a plain, wholesome, and nutritious diet. Their taste is so perverted they have no appetite for a wholesome diet of fruits, plain bread and vegetables. They need not expect to relish at first food so different from that which they have been indulging themselves to eat. {131} If they cannot at first enjoy plain food, they should fast until they can. That fast will prove to them of greater benefit than MEDICINE, for the abused stomach will find that rest which it has long needed, and real hunger can be satisfied with a plain diet. It will take time for the taste to recover from the abuses which it has received, and to gain its natural tone. But perseverance in a self-denying course of eating and drinking will soon make plain, wholesome food palatable, and it will soon be eaten with greater satisfaction than the epicure enjoys over his rich dainties. . . . {133}

(*Counsels on Diet and Foods*, 158–159; *Medical Ministry*, 282; *Testimony Studies on Diet and Foods*, 51, 128.
FP—*Counsels on Health*, 148.)

"I was shown that more deaths have been caused by DRUG TAKING than from all other causes combined. If there was in the land one physician in the place of thousands, a vast amount of premature mortality would be prevented. Multitudes of physicians, and multitudes of DRUGS, have cursed the inhabitants of the earth, and have carried thousands and tens of thousands to untimely graves.

(*Review and Herald,* September 5, 1899; *Selected Messages,* book 2, 450.)

"Indulging in eating too frequently, and in too large quantities, over-taxes the digestive organs, and produces a feverish state of the system. The blood becomes impure, and then diseases of various kinds occur. A physician is sent for, who prescribes some DRUG which gives present relief, but which does not cure the disease. It may change the form of disease, but the real evil is increased tenfold. Nature was doing her best to rid the system of an accumulation of impurities, and could she have been left to herself, aided by the common blessings of Heaven, such as pure air and pure water, a speedy and safe cure would have been ef-fected.

(*Counsels on Diet and Foods,* 304; *Review and Herald,* September 5, 1899; *Medical Ministry,* 281; *Selected Messages,* book 2, 450; *Testimony Studies on Diet and Foods,* 51.*)*

"The sufferers in such cases can do for themselves that which oth-ers cannot do as well for them. They should commence to relieve nature of the load they have forced upon her. They should remove the cause. Fast a short time, and give the stomach chance for rest. Reduce the feverish state of the system by a careful and understanding application of water. These {134} efforts will help nature in her struggles to free the system of impurities. But generally the persons who suffer pain be-come impatient. They are not willing to use self-denial, and suffer a little from hunger. Neither are they willing to wait the slow process of nature to build up the overtaxed energies of the system. But they are deter-mined to obtain relief at once, and take POWERFUL DRUGS, prescribed by physicians. Nature was doing her work well, and would have tri-umphed, but while accomplishing her task, a FOREIGN SUBSTANCE of a POISONOUS NATURE was introduced. What a mistake! Abused nature has now two evils to war against instead of one. She leaves the work in which she was engaged, and resolutely takes hold to expel the intruder newly introduced into the system. Nature feels this double draft upon her resources, and she becomes enfeebled.

(*Selected Messages,* book 2, 450–451; *Review and Herald,* September 5, 1899. MP—*Mind, Character, and Personality,* vol. 2, 512.)

"DRUGS never cure disease. They only change the form and loca-tion. Nature alone is the effectual restorer, and how much better could she perform her task if left to herself. But this privilege is seldom al-lowed her. If crippled nature bears up under the load, and finally accom-plishes in a great measure her double task, and the patient lives, the

credit is given to the physician. But if nature fails in her effort to expel the POISON from the system, and the patient dies, it is called a wonderful dispensation of Providence. If the patient had taken a course to relieve overburdened nature in season, and understandingly used pure soft water, this dispensation of DRUG MORTALITY might have been wholly averted. The use of water can accomplish but little, if the patient does not feel the necessity of also strictly attending to his diet. . . . {135}
(*Review and Herald*, September 5, 1899; *Selected Messages*, book 2, 451.)

"When DRUGS are introduced into the system, for a time they may seem to have a beneficial effect. A change may take place, but the disease is not cured. It will manifest itself in some other form. In nature's efforts to expel the DRUG from the system, intense suffering is sometimes caused the patient. And the disease, which the DRUG was given to cure, may disappear, but only to re-appear in a new form, such as skin diseases, ulcers, painful diseased joints, and sometimes in a more dangerous and deadly form. The liver, heart, and brain, are frequently affected by DRUGS, and often all these organs are burdened with disease, and the unfortunate subjects, if they live, are invalids for life, wearily dragging out a miserable existence. Oh, how much that POISONOUS DRUG cost! If it did not cost the life, it cost quite too much. Nature has been crippled in all her efforts. The whole machinery is out of order, and at a future period in life, when these fine works which have been injured, are to be relied upon to act a more important part in union with all the fine works of nature's machinery, they cannot readily and strongly perform their labor, and the whole system feels the lack. These organs, which should be in a healthy condition, are enfeebled, the blood becomes impure. Nature keeps struggling, and the patient suffers with different ailments, until there is a sudden breaking down in her efforts, and death follows. There are more who die from the use of DRUGS, than all who would have died of disease had nature been left to do her own work.
(*Selected Messages*, book 2, 451–452; *Review and Herald*, September 5, 1899. F & LP—*Healthful Living*, 185, 202, 243–244; *Review and Herald*, April 2, 1914.)

"Very many lives have been sacrificed by physicians' administering DRUGS for unknown diseases. They have no real knowledge of the exact disease which afflicts the patient. But physicians are expected to know in a moment what to do, and unless they act at {136} once as though they understood the disease perfectly, they are considered by impatient friends, and by the sick, as incompetent physicians. Therefore, to gratify erroneous opinions of the sick and their friends, MEDICINE must be administered, experiments and tests tried to cure the patient of the disease of which they have no real knowledge. Nature is loaded with POISONOUS DRUGS which she cannot expel from the system. The physicians themselves are often convinced that they have used POWERFUL MEDICINES for a disease which did not exist, and death was the consequence. (*Selected Messages,* book 2, 452; *Review and Herald,* September 5, 1899.)

"Physicians are censurable, but they are not the only ones at fault. The sick themselves, if they would be patient, diet and suffer a little, and give nature time to rally, would recover much sooner without the use of ANY MEDICINE. Nature alone possesses curative powers. MEDICINES have no power to cure, but will most generally hinder nature in her efforts. She after all must do the work of restoring. The sick are in a hurry to get well, and the friends of the sick are impatient. They will have MEDICINE, and if they do not feel that powerful influence upon their systems, their erroneous views lead them to think they should feel, they impatiently change for another physician. The change often increases the evil. They go through a course of MEDICINE equally as dangerous as the first, and more fatal, because the two treatments do not agree, and the system is poisoned beyond remedy. . . . {137} (*Review and Herald,* September 12, 1899; *Selected Messages,* book 2, 452–453. MP—*Healthful Living,* 244; *Temperance,* 83. LP—*Healthful Living,* 245.)

"Multitudes remain in inexcusable ignorance in regard to the laws of their being. They are wondering why our race is so feeble, and why so many die prematurely. Is there not a cause? Physicians who profess to understand the human organism, prescribe for their patients, and even for their own dear children, and their companions, SLOW POISONS to break up disease, or to cure slight indisposition. Surely, they cannot realize the evil of these things as they were presented before me, or they could not do thus. The effects of the POISON may not be immediately perceived, but it is doing its work surely in the system, undermining the constitution, and crippling nature in her efforts. They are seeking to correct an evil, but produce a far greater one, which is often incurable. Those who are thus dealt with are constantly sick, and constantly dosing. And yet, if you listen to their conversation, you will often hear them praising the DRUGS they have been using, and recommending their use to others, because they have been benefited by their use. It would seem that to such as can reason from cause to effect, the sallow countenance, the continual complaints of ailments and general prostration of those who claim to be benefited, would be sufficient proofs of the health-destroying influence of DRUGS. And yet many are so blinded they do not see that all the DRUGS they have taken have not cured them, but made them worse. The DRUG INVALID numbers one in the world, but is generally peevish, irritable, always sick, lingering out a miserable existence, and seems to live only to call into constant exercise the patience of others. POISON-OUS DRUGS have not killed them outright, for nature is loath to give up her hold on life. She is unwilling to cease her struggles. Yet these DRUG TAKERS are never well. They are always taking cold, which causes extreme {138} suffering, because of the POISON all through their system.

(FP—*Review and Herald,* September 12, 1899; *Selected Messages,* book 2, 453-454.)

"A branch was presented before me bearing large flat seeds. Upon it was written, NUX VOMICA, STRYCHNINE. Beneath was written, No antidote. I was shown persons under the influence of this POISON. It produced heat, and seemed to act particularly on the spinal column, but affected the whole system. When this is taken in the smallest quantities, it has its influence, which nothing can counteract. If taken immoderately, convulsions, paralysis, insanity, and death, are often the results. Many use this deadly evil in small quantities. But if they realized its influence, not one grain of it would be introduced into the system.

"When first taken, its influence may seem to be beneficial. It excites the nerves connected with the spinal column, but when the excitement passes away, it is followed by a sense of prostration and of chilliness the whole length of the spinal column, especially upon the head and back of the neck. The patients generally cannot endure the least draught of air. They are inclined to close every crevice, and for want of the free, invigorating air of heaven, the blood becomes impure, the vital organs are weakened, and general debility is the result. By unduly exciting the sensitive nerves connected with the spinal column, by this POISONOUS DRUG, they lose their tone and vitality, and weakness of the back and limbs follows. The sight and hearing are often affected, and in many cases the patient becomes helpless.

"I was shown that the innocent, modest-looking, white poppy yields a DANGEROUS DRUG. OPIUM is a SLOW POISON, when taken in small quantities. In large doses it produces lethargy and death. Its effects upon the nervous system are ruinous. When patients use this DRUG until it becomes habit, it is almost impossible to discontinue it, because they feel so prostrated and nervous without it. They are in a worse condition when deprived of it than the RUM DRINKER without his RUM, or the TOBACCO USER deprived of his TOBACCO. {139} The OPIUM SLAVE is in a pitiful condition. Unless his nervous system is continually intoxicated with the POISONOUS DRUG, he is miserable. It benumbs the sensibilities, stupefies the brain, and unfits the mind for the service of God. True Christians cannot persist in the use of this SLOW POISON, when they know its influence upon them.

"Those who use OPIUM cannot render to God any more acceptable service than can the drunkard, or the TOBACCO USER. Those who break off the use of this nerve and brain-destroying practice will have to possess fortitude, and suffer, as will the drunkard, and the TOBACCO SLAVE, when deprived of their body and mind-destroying indulgences. God is displeased that his followers should become slaves to habits which ruin body and mind. NUX VOMICA, or STRYCHNINE, and OPIUM have killed their millions, and have left thousands upon the earth to linger out a wretched, suffering existence, a burden to themselves, and those around them.

"MERCURY, CALOMEL, and QUININE have brought their amount of wretchedness, which the day of God alone will fully reveal. Preparations of MERCURY and CALOMEL taken into the system ever retain their poisonous strength as long as there is a particle of it left in the system. These POISONOUS PREPARATIONS have destroyed their millions, and left sufferers upon the earth to linger out a miserable existence. All are better off without these DANGEROUS MIXTURES. Miserable sufferers, with disease in almost every form, misshapen by suffering, with dreadful ulcers, and pains in the bones, loss of teeth, loss of memory, and impaired sight, are to be seen almost everywhere. They are victims of POISONOUS PREPARATIONS, which have been, in many cases, administered to cure some slight indisposition, which after a day or two of fasting would have disappeared without MEDICINE. But POISONOUS MIXTURES, administered by physicians, have proved their ruin.

"The endless variety of MEDICINES in the market, the numerous advertisements of new DRUGS and MIXTURES, all of which, as they say, do wonderful cures, kill {140} hundreds where they benefit one. Those who are sick are not patient. They will take the various MEDICINES, some of which are very powerful, although they know nothing of the nature of the MIXTURES. All the MEDICINES they take only make their recovery more hopeless. Yet they keep dosing, and continue to

grow weaker, until they die. Some will have MEDICINE at all events. Then let them take these HURTFUL MIXTURES and the various DEADLY POISONS upon their own responsibility. God's servants should not administer MEDICINES which they know will leave behind injurious effects upon the system, even if they do relieve present suffering.
(*Healthful Living,* 245; LP—*Selected Messages,* book 2, 281; *Temperance, 87.*)

"Every POISONOUS PREPARATION in the vegetable and mineral kingdoms, taken into the system, will leave its wretched influence, affecting the liver and lungs, and deranging the system generally. Nor does the evil end here. Diseased, feeble infants are brought into the world to share this misery, transmitted to them from their parents.
(FP—*Selected Messages,* book 2, 454; *Healthful Living,* 245; *Temperance,* 87;
MP—*Selected Messages,* book 2, 281; *Healthful Living,* 176.)

"I have been shown that a great amount of suffering might be saved if all would labor to prevent disease, by strictly obeying the laws of health. Strict habits of cleanliness should be observed. Many, while well, will not take the trouble to keep in a healthy condition. They neglect personal cleanliness, and are not careful to keep their clothing pure. Impurities are constantly and imperceptibly passing from the body, through the pores of the skin, and if the surface of the skin is not kept in a healthy condition, the system is burdened with impure matter. If the clothing worn is not often washed, and frequently aired, it becomes filthy with impurities which are thrown off from the body by sensible and insensible perspiration. And if the garments worn are not frequently cleansed from these impurities, the pores of the skin absorb again the waste matter thrown off. The impurities of the body, if not allowed to escape, are taken back into the blood, and forced upon the internal organs. Nature, to relieve herself of poisonous impurities, makes an effort to free the {141} system, which effort produces fevers, and what is termed disease. But even then, if those who are afflicted would assist nature in her efforts, by the use of pure, soft water, much suffering would be prevented. But many, instead of doing this, and seeking to remove the poisonous matter from the system, take a more DEADLY POISON into the system, to remove a poison already there. . . . {145}

"Those who will gratify their appetite, and then suffer because of their intemperance, and take DRUGS to relieve them, may be assured that God will not interpose to save health and life which is so recklessly periled. The cause has produced the effect. Many, as their last resort, follow the directions in the Word of God, and request the prayers of the

Spirit of Prophecy References

elders of the church for their restoration to health. God does not see fit to answer prayers offered in behalf of such, for he knows that if they should be restored to health, they would again sacrifice it upon the altar of unhealthy appetite.

(*Counsels on Diet and Foods,* 26; *Medical Ministry,* 14; *Testimony Studies on Diet and Foods,* 185–186.)

"There is a class of invalids who have no real located disease. But as they believe they are dangerously diseased, they are in reality invalids. The mind is diseased, and many die who might recover of disease, which exists alone in the imagination. If such could have their minds diverted from themselves, from noticing every poor feeling, they would soon improve. Inactivity will cause disease. And to this the indulgence of unhealthy appetite, and DRUGTAKING, and those who had no real located disease will become invalids in very deed. They make themselves so. If such would engage in cheerful, healthy labor, they would rise above poor feelings. Even if they should become very weary at times it would not hurt them. As they would accustom themselves to healthy, active labor, the mind would be occupied, and not find time to dwell upon every ache and pain.

"If invalids would dispense with MEDICINES of every description, and improve their habits of eating, and exercise as much as possible in the open air, their names would soon be dropped from the invalid list. The power of the will is a mighty soother of the nerves, and can resist much disease, simply by not yielding to ailments, and settling down into a state of inactivity. Those who have but little force, and {146} natural energy, need to constantly guard themselves, lest their minds become diseased, and they give up to supposed disease, when none really exists. It is slow murder for persons to confine themselves days, weeks and months indoors, with but little outdoor exercise."

1864—*Spiritual Gifts,* vol. 4A, 152–153.

"We expected the crisis would come the seventh day. We had but little rest during his sickness, and were obliged to give him up into others' care the fourth and fifth nights. My husband and myself the fifth day felt very anxious. The child raised fresh blood, and coughed considerably. My husband spent much time in prayer. We left our child in careful hands that night. Before retiring my husband prayed long and earnestly. Suddenly his burden of prayer left him, and it seemed as though a voice spoke to him, and said, Go lie down, I will take care of the child. I had retired sick, and could not sleep for anxiety for several hours. I felt pressed for breath. Although sleeping in a large chamber, I arose and opened the door into a large hall, and was at once relieved, and soon slept. I dreamed that an experienced physician was standing by my child, watching every breath, with one hand over his heart, and with the other feeling his pulse. He turned to us and said, 'The crisis has passed. He has seen his worst night. He will now come up speedily, for he has not the injurious influence of DRUGS to recover from. Nature has nobly done her work to rid the system of impurities.' I related to him my worn-out condition, my pressure for breath, and the relief obtained by opening the door. Said he, 'That which gave you relief, will also relieve your child. He needs air. You have kept him too warm. The heated air coming from a stove is injurious, and were it not for the air coming in at the crevices of the windows, would be poisonous, and destroy life. Stove heat destroys the vitality of the air, and weakens the lungs. The child's lungs have been weakened by the room being kept too warm. Sick persons are debilitated by disease, and need all the invigorating air that they can bear to strengthen the vital organs to resist disease. And yet in most cases air and light are excluded from the sick room at the {153} very time when most needed, as though dangerous enemies.' "

(MP—*Selected Messages*, book 2, 305; *Pamphlet 144, The Place of Herbs in Rational Therapy*, 21; *The Ellen G. White Biography*, 1862, vol. 2, 78)

1865—*Review and Herald*, December 5, 1899.

"In no case should sick persons be deprived of a full supply of fresh air in pleasant weather. Their rooms may not always be so constructed as to allow the windows or doors to be opened, without the draft coming directly upon them, thus exposing them to the taking of cold. In such cases windows and doors should be opened in an adjoining room, thus letting fresh air enter the room occupied by the sick. Fresh air will prove far more beneficial to sick persons than MEDICINE and is far more essential to them than their food. They will do better and will recover sooner when deprived of food than when deprived of fresh air.

(*Counsels on Health*, 55.)

"Many invalids have been confined for weeks and even for months in close rooms, with the light, and the pure, invigorating air of heaven shut out as if air were a deadly enemy, when it was just the MEDICINE they needed to make them well. The whole system was debilitated and diseased for want of air, and nature sank under her load of accumulating impurities, in addition to the FASHIONABLE POISONS administered by physicians, until she was overpowered, and broke down in her efforts, and death was the

result. These persons might have lived. Heaven willed not their death. They died, victims to their own ignorance and the deception of physicians, who gave them FASHIONABLE POISONS, and would not allow them pure water to drink, and fresh air to breathe, to invigorate the vital organs, purify the blood, and help nature in her task in overcoming the bad conditions of the system. These valuable remedies which Heaven has provided, without money and without price, were cast aside, and considered not only as worthless, but even as dangerous enemies, while POISONS, prescribed by physicians, were in blind confidence taken."
(*Counsels on Health*, 55)

1865—*Healthful Living*, 244, 246.

"Sick people who take DRUGS do appear to get well. With some there is sufficient life force for nature to draw upon to so far expel the POISON from the system that the sick, having a period of rest, recover. But no credit should be allowed the DRUGS taken, for they only hindered nature in her efforts. All the credit should be ascribed to nature's restorative powers. . . .{246}

"Everywhere you go you will see deformity, disease, and imbecility, which in very many cases can be traced directly back to DRUG POISONS."

1865—*Selected Messages*, book 2, 441–450, 453–454.

"The human family have brought upon themselves diseases of various forms by their own wrong habits. They have not studied how to live healthfully, and their transgression of the laws of their being has produced a deplorable state of things. The people have seldom accredited their sufferings to the true cause—their own wrong course of action. They have indulged an intemperance in eating, and made a god of their appetite. In all their habits they have manifested a recklessness in regard to health and life; and when, as the result, sickness has come upon them they have made themselves believe that God was the author of it, when their own wrong course of action has brought the sure result. When in distress they send for the doctor, and trust their bodies in his hands, expecting that he will make them well. He deals out to them DRUGS, the nature of which they know nothing, and in their blind confidence they swallow anything that the doctor may choose to give. Thus POWERFUL POISONS are often administered which fetter nature in all her friendly efforts to recover the abuse the system has suffered, and the patient is hurried out of this life. . . .
(*Review and Herald*, August 15, 1899)

Spirit of Prophecy References

"He makes the case a grave one, and administers his POISONS, which, if he were sick, he would not venture to take himself. The patient grows worse, and POISONOUS DRUGS are more freely administered, until nature is overpowered in her efforts, and gives up the conflict, and the {442} mother dies. She was DRUGGED to death. Her system was poisoned beyond remedy. She was murdered. Neighbors and relatives marvel at the wonderful dealings of Providence in thus removing a mother in the midst of her usefulness, at the period when her children need her care so much. They wrong our good and wise Heavenly Father when they cast back upon Him this weight of human woe. Heaven wished that mother to live, and her untimely death dishonored God. The mother's wrong habits, and her inattention to the laws of her being, made her sick. And the doctor's FASHIONABLE POISONS, introduced into the system, closed the period of her existence, and left a helpless, stricken, motherless flock.

(*Review and Herald,* August 15, 1899)

"The above is not always the result which follows the doctor's DRUGGING. Sick people who take these DRUG POISONS do appear to get well. With some, there is sufficient life force for nature to draw upon, to so far expel the POISON from the system that the sick, having a period of rest, recover. But no credit should be allowed the DRUGS taken, for they only hindered nature in her efforts. All the credit should be ascribed to nature's restorative powers.

(*Review and Herald,* August 15, 1899)

"Although the patient may recover, yet the powerful effort nature was required to make to induce action to overcome the POISON, injured the constitution, and shortened the life of the patient. There are many who do not die under the influence of DRUGS, but there are very many who are left useless wrecks, hopeless, gloomy, and miserable sufferers, a burden to themselves and to society.

(*Review and Herald,* August 15, 1899; *Healthful Living,* 245)

"If those who take these DRUGS were alone the sufferers, then the evil would not be as great. But parents not only sin against themselves in swallowing DRUG POISONS, but they sin against their children. The vitiated state of their blood, the POISON distributed throughout the system, the broken constitution, and various DRUG DISEASES, as the result of DRUG POISONS, are transmitted to their offspring, and left them as a wretched inheritance, which is another great cause of the degeneracy of the race.

Spirit of Prophecy References

(*Review and Herald,* August 15, 1899; *Temperance,* 84–85)
LP—*Healthful Living,* 57)

"Physicians, by administering their DRUG POISONS, have done very much to increase the depreciation of the race, physically, mentally, and morally. Everywhere you may go you will see deformity, disease and imbecility, which in very many cases can be traced directly back to the DRUG POISONS, administered by the hand of a doctor, as a remedy for some of life's ills. The so-called remedy has fearfully {443} proved itself to the patient, by stern suffering experience, to be far worse than the disease for which the DRUG was taken. All who possess common capabilities should understand the wants of their own system. The philosophy of health should compose one of the important studies for our children. It is all-important that the human organism be understood, and then intelligent men and women can be their own physicians. If the people would reason from cause to effect, and would follow the light which shines upon them, they would pursue a course which would insure health, and mortality would be far less. But the people are too willing to remain in inexcusable ignorance, and trust their bodies to the doctors, instead of having any special responsibility in the matter themselves. . . .
(*Review and Herald,* August 15, 1899)

"The physician then inquired in regard to the nature and length of the sickness of those who had died. The father moanfully related the painful facts connected with the illness of his loved ones. 'My son was first attacked with a fever. I called a physician. He said that he could administer MEDICINE which would soon break the fever. He gave him POWERFUL MEDICINE, but was disappointed in its effects. The fever was reduced, but my son grew dangerously sick. The same MEDICINE was again given him, without producing any change for the better. The physician then resorted to still more POWERFUL MEDICINES, but my son obtained no relief. The fever left him, but he did not rally. He sank rapidly and died.

"The death of my son so sudden and unexpected was a great grief to us all, but especially to his mother. Her watching and anxiety in his sickness, and her grief occasioned by his sudden death, were too much for her nervous system, {444} and my wife was soon prostrated. I felt dissatisfied with the course pursued by this physician. My confidence in his skill was shaken, and I could not employ him a second time. I called another to my suffering wife. This second physician gave her a liberal dose of OPIUM, which he said would relieve her pains, quiet her nerves,

and give her rest, which she much needed. The OPIUM stupefied her. She slept, and nothing could arouse her from the deathlike stupor. Her pulse and heart at times throbbed violently, and then grew more and more feeble in their action, until she ceased to breathe. Thus she died without giving her family one look of recognition. This second death seemed more than we could endure. We all sorrowed deeply but I was agonized and could not be comforted. . . .
(*Review and Herald,* August 15, 1899)

"This third physician professed to understand my daughter's case. He said that she was greatly debilitated, and that her nervous system was deranged, and that fever was upon her, which could be controlled, but that it would take time to bring her up from her present state of debility. He expressed perfect confidence in his ability to raise her. He gave her POWERFUL MEDICINE to break up the fever. This was accomplished. But as the fever left, the case assumed more alarming features, and grew more complicated. As the symptoms changed, the MEDICINES were varied to meet the case. While under the influence of new MEDICINES she would, for a time, appear revived, which would flatter our hopes, that she would get well, only to make our disappointment more bitter as she became worse.
(*Review and Herald,* August 15, 1899)

"The physician's last resort was CALOMEL. For some time she seemed to be between life and death. She was thrown into convulsions. As these most distressing spasms ceased, we were aroused to the painful fact that her intellect was weakened. She began slowly to improve, although still a great sufferer. Her limbs were crippled as the effect of the POWERFUL POISONS which she had taken. She lingered a few years a helpless, pitiful sufferer, and died in much agony. . . . {445}
(*Review and Herald,* August 15, 1899)

"Another scene was then presented before me. I was brought into the presence of a female, apparently about thirty years of age. A physician was standing by her, and reporting, that her nervous system was deranged, that her blood was impure, and moved sluggishly, and that her stomach was in a cold, inactive condition. He said that he would give her active remedies which would soon improve her condition. He gave her a powder from a vial upon which was written, NUX VOMICA. I watched to see what effect this would have upon the patient. It appeared to act favorably. Her condition seemed better. She was animated, and even seemed cheerful and active.

"My attention was then called to still another case. I was intro-

duced into the sick room of a young man who was in a high fever. A physician was standing by the bedside of the sufferer with a portion of MEDICINE taken from a vial upon which was written CALOMEL. He administered this chemical POISON, and a change seemed to take place, but not for the better.
(*Review and Herald,* August 22, 1899)

"I was then shown still another case. It was that of a female, who seemed to be suffering much pain. A physician stood by the bedside of the patient, and was administering MEDICINE, taken from a vial, upon which was written, OPIUM. At first this DRUG seemed to affect the mind. She talked strangely, but finally became quiet and slept.
(*Review and Herald,* August 22, 1899)

"My attention was then called to the first case, that of the father who had lost his wife and two children. The physician was in the sick room, standing by the bedside of the afflicted daughter. Again he left the room without giving MEDICINE. The father, when in the presence of the physician alone seemed deeply moved, and he inquired impatiently, 'Do you intend to do nothing? Will you leave my only daughter to die?' The physician said—
(*Review and Herald,* August 22, 1899)

" 'I have listened to the sad history of the death of your much loved wife, and your two children, and have learned from your own lips that all three have died while in the care of physicians, while taking MEDICINES prescribed and administered by their hands. MEDICINE has not saved your {446} loved ones, and as a physician I solemnly believe that none of them need, or ought to have died. They could have recovered if they had not been so DRUGGED that nature was enfeebled by abuse, and finally crushed.' He stated decidedly to the agitated father 'I cannot give MEDICINE to your daughter. I shall only seek to assist nature in her efforts, by removing every obstruction, and then leave nature to recover the exhausted energies of the system.' He placed in the father's hand a few directions which he enjoined upon him to follow closely. . . .
(*Review and Herald,* August 22, 1899)

"The father looked sad and doubtful, but submitted to the decision of the physician. He feared that his daughter must die if she had no MEDICINE.
(*Review and Herald,* August 22, 1899)

"The second case was again presented before me. The patient had appeared better under the influence of NUX VOMICA. She was sitting up, folding a shawl closely around her, and complaining of chilliness. The

air in the room was impure. It was heated and had lost its vitality. Almost every crevice where pure air could enter was guarded, to protect the patient from a sense of painful chilliness, which was especially felt in the back of the neck and down the spinal column. If the door was left ajar, she seemed nervous and distressed, and entreated that it should be closed, for she was cold. She could not bear the least draft of air from the door or windows. A gentleman of {447} intelligence stood looking pityingly upon her, and said to those present—
(Review and Herald, August 22, 1899)

" 'This is the second result of NUX VOMICA. It is especially felt upon the nerves, and it affects the whole nervous system. There will be, for a time, increased forced action upon the nerves. But as the strength of this DRUG is spent, there will be chilliness and prostration. Just to the degree that it excites and enlivens will be the deadening, benumbing results following.'
(Review and Herald, August 22, 1899)

"The third case was again presented before me. It was that of the young man to whom was administered CALOMEL. He was a great sufferer. His lips were dark and swollen. His gums were inflamed. His tongue was thick and swollen, and the saliva was running from his mouth in large quantities. The intelligent gentleman before mentioned looked sadly upon the sufferer, and said—
(Review and Herald, August 22, 1899)

" 'This is the influence of MERCURIAL PREPARATIONS. This young man had remaining, sufficient nervous energy, to commence a warfare upon this intruder, this DRUG POISON to attempt to expel it from the system. Many have not sufficient life-forces left to arouse to action, and nature is overpowered and ceases her efforts, and the victim dies.'
(Review and Herald, August 22, 1899)

"The fourth case, the person to whom was given OPIUM, was again presented before me. She had awakened from her sleep much prostrated. Her mind was distracted. She was impatient and irritable, finding fault with her best friends, and imagining that they did not try to relieve her sufferings. She became frantic, and raved like a maniac. The gentleman before mentioned looked sadly upon the sufferer, and said to those present—
(Review and Herald, August 29, 1899)

" 'This is the second result from taking OPIUM.' Her physician was called. He gave her an increased dose of OPIUM which quieted her ravings, yet made her very talkative and cheerful. She was at peace with all around her, and expressed much affection for acquaintances, as well as her relatives. She soon grew drowsy and fell into a stupefied condition. The gentleman mentioned above, solemnly said—

(*Review and Herald*, August 29, 1899)

" 'Her conditions of health are no better now than when she was in her frantic ravings. She is decidedly worse. This DRUG POISON, OPIUM, gives temporary relief from pain, but does not remove the cause of pain. It only stupefies the brain, rendering it incapable of receiving impressions from the nerves. While the brain is thus insensible, the hearing, {448} the taste, and sight are affected. When the influence of OPIUM wears off, and the brain arouses from its state of paralysis, the nerves, which had been cut off from communication with the brain, shriek out louder than ever the pains in the system, because of the additional outrage the system has sustained in receiving this POISON. Every additional DRUG given to the patient, whether it be OPIUM, or some other POISON, will complicate the case, and make the patient's recovery more hopeless. The DRUGS given to stupefy, whatever they may be, derange the nervous system. An evil, simple in the beginning, which nature aroused herself to overcome, and which she would have done had she been left to herself, has been made tenfold worse by DRUG POISONS being introduced into the system, which is a destructive disease of itself, forcing into extraordinary action the remaining life forces to war against and overcome the DRUG INTRUDER.'

(*Review and Herald*, August 29, 1899;
MP—*Healthful Living*, 195, 202; *Temperance*, 83; *Healthful Living*, 202; LP—*Healthful Living*, 243-244)

"I was brought again into the sickroom of the first case, that of the father and his daughter. The daughter was sitting by the side of her father, cheerful and happy, with the glow of health upon her countenance. The father was looking upon her with happy satisfaction, his countenance speaking the gratitude of his heart, that his only child was spared to him. Her physician entered, and after conversing with the father and child for a short time, arose to leave. He addressed the father, thus—

" 'I present to you your daughter restored to health. I gave her no MEDICINE that I might leave her with an unbroken constitution. MEDICINE never could have accomplished this. MEDICINE deranges nature's fine machinery, and breaks down the constitution, and kills, but never cures. Nature alone possesses the restorative powers. She alone can build up her exhausted energies, and repair the injuries she has received by inat-

tention to her fixed laws.'
(*Review and Herald,* August 29, 1899;
MP—*Healthful Living,* 244.)

"He then asked the father if he was satisfied with his manner of treatment. The happy father expressed his heartfelt gratitude, and perfect satisfaction, saying—

" 'I have learned a lesson I shall never forget. It was painful, yet it is of priceless value. I am now convinced that my wife and children need not have died. Their lives were sacrificed while in the hands of physicians by their POISONOUS DRUGS.'
(*Review and Herald,* August 29, 1899;
FP—*Healthful Living,* 202.)

"I was then shown the second case, the patient to {449} whom NUX VOMICA had been administered. She was being supported by two attendants, from her chair to her bed. She had nearly lost the use of her limbs. The spinal nerves were partially paralyzed, and the limbs had lost their power to bear the weight of the person. She coughed distressingly, and breathed with difficulty. She was laid upon the bed, and soon lost her hearing, and seeing, and thus she lingered awhile, and died. The gentleman before mentioned looked sorrowfully upon the lifeless body, and said to those present—
(*Review and Herald,* August 29, 1899)

" 'Witness the mildest and protracted influence of NUX VOMICA upon the human system. At its introduction, the nervous energy was excited to extraordinary action to meet this DRUG POISON. This extra excitement was followed by prostration, and the final result has been paralysis of the nerves. This DRUG does not have the same effect upon all. Some who have powerful constitutions can recover from abuses to which they may subject the system. While others, whose hold of life is not as strong, who possess enfeebled constitutions, have never recovered from receiving into the system even one dose, and many die from no other cause than the effects of one portion of this POISON. Its effects are always tending to death. The condition the system is in, at the time these POISONS are received into it, determine the life of the patient. NUX VOMICA can cripple, paralyze, destroy health forever, but it never cures.'
(*Review and Herald,* August 29, 1899;
FP—*Healthful Living,* 202.)

"The third case was again presented before me, that of the young man to whom had been administered CALOMEL. He was a pitiful sufferer. His limbs were crippled, and he was greatly deformed. He stated

that his sufferings were beyond description, and life was to him a great burden. The gentleman whom I have repeatedly mentioned, looked upon the sufferer with sadness and pity, and said—
(*Review and Herald*, August 29, 1899)

" 'This is the effect of CALOMEL. It torments the system as long as there is a particle left in it. It ever lives, not losing its properties by its long stay in the living system. It inflames the joints, and often sends rottenness into the bones. It frequently manifests itself in tumors, ulcers, and cancers, years after it has been introduced into the system.'
(*Review and Herald*, August 29, 1899; F & LP—*Healthful Living*, 190)

"The fourth case was again presented before me—the patient to whom OPIUM had been administered. Her countenance was sallow, and her eyes were restless and glassy. Her hands shook as if palsied, and she seemed to be greatly {450} excited, imagining that all present were leagued against her. Her mind was a complete wreck, and she raved in a pitiful manner. The physician was summoned, and seemed to be unmoved at these terrible exhibitions. He gave the patient a more POWERFUL POR-TION of OPIUM, which he said would set her all right. Her ravings did not cease until she became thoroughly intoxicated. She then passed into a deathlike stupor. The gentleman mentioned, looked upon the patient, and said sadly—
(*Review and Herald*, August 29, 1899)

" 'Her days are numbered. The efforts nature has made have been so many times overpowered by this POISON, that the vital forces are exhausted by being repeatedly induced to unnatural action to rid the system of this POISONOUS DRUG. Nature's efforts are about to cease, and then the patient's suffering life will end.'
(*Review and Herald*, August 29, 1899)

"More deaths have been caused by DRUG TAKING than from all other causes combined. If there was in the land one physician in the place of thousands, a vast amount of premature mortality would be prevented. Multitudes of physicians, and multitudes of DRUGS, have cursed the inhabitants of the earth, and have carried thousands and tens of thousands to untimely graves. . . . {453}
(*Review and Herald*, September 5, 1899)

"Multitudes remain in inexcusable ignorance in regard to the laws of their being. They are wondering why our race is so feeble, and why so many die prematurely. Is there not a cause? Physicians who profess to understand the human organism, prescribe for their patients, and even for their own dear children, and their companions, SLOW POISONS to break up disease, or to cure slight indisposition. Surely, they cannot realize the evil of these things or they could not do thus. The effects of the POISON may not be immediately perceived, but it is doing its work surely in the system, undermining the constitution, and crippling nature in her efforts. They are seeking to correct an evil, but produce a far greater one, which is often incurable. Those who are thus dealt with, are constantly sick, and constantly dosing. And yet, if you listen to their conversation, you will often hear them praising the DRUGS they have been using, and recommending their use to others, because {454} they have been benefited by their use. It would seem that to such as can reason from cause to effect, the sallow countenance, the continual complaints of ailments, and general prostration of those who claim to be benefited, would be suffieient proofs of the health-destroying influence of DRUGS. And yet many are so blinded they do not see that all the DRUGS they have taken have not cured them, but made them worse. The DRUG INVALID numbers one in the world, but is generally peevish, irritable, always sick, lingering out a miserable existence, and seems to live only to call into constant exercise the patience of others. POISONOUS DRUGS have not killed them outright, for nature is loath to give up her hold on life. She is unwilling to cease her struggles. Yet these DRUG TAKERS are never well."

(*Review and Herald,* September 12, 1899)

1865—*Selected Messages,* book 2, 455—456.

"In pleasant weather the sick in no case should be deprived of a full supply of fresh air. Their rooms may not always be so constructed as to allow the windows or doors open in their rooms, without the draught coming directly {456} upon them, and exposing them to take cold. In such cases windows and doors should be opened in an adjoining room and thus let the fresh air enter the room occupied by the sick. Fresh air will prove more beneficial to the sick than MEDICINE, and is far more essential to them than their food. They will do better, and recover sooner, deprived of food, than of fresh air.

(*Healthful Living,* 157)

"Many invalids have been confined weeks and months in close rooms, shutting out the light, and pure, invigorating air of heaven, as though air was a deadly enemy, when it was just the MEDICINE the sick needed to make them well. The whole system was debilitated and diseased for want of air, and nature was sinking under her load of accumulating impurities, in addition to the FASHIONABLE POISONS administered by physicians, until she was overpowered, and broke down in her efforts, and the sick died. They might have lived. Heaven willed not their death. They died victims to their own ignorance, and that of their frineds, and the ignorance and deception of physicians, who gave them fashionable poisons, and would not allow them pure water to drink, and fresh air to breathe, to invigorate the vital organs, purify the blood, and help nature in her task in overcoming the bad conditions of the system. These valuable remedies which Heaven has provided, without money and without price, were cast aside, and considered not only as worthless, but even as dangerous enemies, while POISONS, prescribed by physicians, were in blind confidence taken.

(*Review and Herald*, December 5, 1899)

"Thousands have died for want of pure water and pure air, who might have lived. And thousands of living invalids, who are a burden to themselves and others, think that their lives depend upon taking MEDICINES from the doctors. They are continually guarding themselves against the air, and avoiding the use of water. These blessings they need in order to become well. If they would become enlightened, and let MEDICINE alone, and accustom themselves to outdoor exercise, and to air in their houses, summer and winter, and use soft water for drinking and bathing purposes, they would be comparatively well and happy, instead of dragging out a miserable existence."

(*Review and Herald*, December 5, 1899; *Counsels on Health*, 55–56; F & LP—*Counsels on Diet and Foods*, 419; *Healthful Living*, 155–156; *Testimony Studies on Diet and Foods*, 151)

1865—*Selected Messages*, book 2, 468.

"When the limbs and arms are chilled, the blood is driven from these parts to the lungs and head. The circulation is impeded, and nature's fine machinery does not move harmoniously. The system of the infant is deranged, and it cries and mourns because of the abuse it is compelled to suffer. The mother feeds it, thinking it must be hungry, when food only increases its suffering. Tight bands and an overloaded stomach do not agree. It has no room to breathe. It may scream, struggle and pant for breath, and yet the mother not mistrust the cause. She could relieve the sufferer at once, at least of tight bandages, if she understood the nature of the case. She at length becomes alarmed, and thinks her child really ill, and summons a doctor, who looks gravely upon the infant a few moments and then deals out POISONOUS MEDICINES, or something called a SOOTHING CORDIAL, which the mother, faithful to directions, pours down the throat of the abused infant. If it was not diseased in reality before, it is after this process. It suffers now from DRUG DISEASE, the most stubborn and incurable of all diseases. If it recovers, it must bear about more or less in its system the effects of that POISONOUS DRUG, and it is liable to spasms, heart disease, dropsy on the brain, or consumption. Some infants are not strong enough to bear even a trifle of DRUG POISONS, and as nature rallies to meet the intruder, the vital forces of the tender infant are too severely taxed, and death ends the scene."

(*The Health Reformer,* January 1, 1872; *Review and Herald,* January 2, 1900; LP—*Healthful Living,* 202)

1866—*Review and Herald,* February 20, 1866.

"We had confidence in the use of water as one of God's appointed remedies, but no confidence in DRUGS. My vital energies were too much exhausted for me to attempt to use water in my husband's case. His wearing labors had long been bringing about the result, and could we expect God to work a miracle to heal him without our using the means or agencies He had provided for us? As there was no one in Battle Creek who dared take the responsibility of administering water in my husband's case, we felt that it might be duty to take him to Dansville, N. Y., where he could rest, and water be applied by those well skilled in its use. We dared not to follow our own judgment. We asked counsel of God, and after a prayerful consideration of the matter decided to go. My husband endured the journey well—much better than we had feared."

Review and Herald, April 16, 1914; *Life Sketches of Ellen G. White,* 169.

1866—*The Health Reformer,* September 1, 1866.

"There is a disposition with many parents, to keep up a perpetual dosing of their children with MEDICINES. They will always have a supply on hand, and when any slight indisposition is manifested, caused by overeating or exhaustion, the MEDICINE is poured down their throats; and if that does not satisfy them, they send for the doctor. If he is an honest physician, and declines to give the child MEDICINE because he is wise enough to know it will be for its hurt, the parents are offended and think the physician inefficient, and send for another, who is less conscientious, and who will give MEDICINE to satisfy the parents, who were blinded by ignorance in regard to the real condition and need of their child. And not unfrequently parents are so anxious to do all they can to save their child, that they change physicians, having two or three to attend the same case. The child is DRUGGED to death, and the parents console themselves that they have done all they could, and wonder why it must die when they did so much to save it. Upon the grave stone of that child should be written, Died, of DRUG MEDICATION.

(F & LP—*Healthful Living*, 149–150)

"Many parents substitute DRUGS for judicious nursing. I have seen parents in constant terror, lest a breath of air should come upon their children. They place them perhaps in a crib or cradle near a hot stove. Their faces are red from heat, and they are pressed for air, and almost gasping for breath. But the mother does not seem to understand their wants. She thinks her children sick, and runs for a CORDIAL which only stupefies them, but makes them no better. The only CORDIAL the suffocated, suffering innocent needed, was pure, fresh air. Several instances have come under my notice, where children were being murdered by inches by the mistaken kindness of parents. They deprived them of air as though it were a DEADLY POISON. The rich blessing which Heaven has freely bestowed upon all, was not allowed to come to their children. I have stood by the cradle of these abused innocents thus unwisely nursed, and have felt indignant at the cruel course pursued with them. I have stripped the coverings from the cradle, and opened the window, and let in the richest of heaven's earthly blessing—pure, fresh air—to the immediate relief of the sufferers.

(FP—*Temperance*, 85; *Healthful Living*, 243)

"Children also are fed too frequently, which produces fever and suffering in various ways. The stomach should not be kept constantly at work; it should have its periods of rest. Without it, children will be peevish and irritable, and frequently sick. The parents do not trace the existing effect to the true cause—a transgression on their part—but hasten for a doctor, expecting that he will set things all right. The mother abuses the laws which govern that child's life, and then commits another transgression by interfering with nature in introducing POISONOUS DRUGS into the system. Children who might have retained a good constitution, are destroyed for lack of knowledge. Many die prematurely, and others live to be lifelong sufferers, a burden to themselves and to society. Who is to blame for all this weight of evil? not our kind Creator surely, for He does not take pleasure in seeing His creatures suffer. He wishes them to be healthful and happy. The parents and physicians are the instruments who have caused this weight of woe. They were ignorant of the terrible wake they left behind them. Ignorance is sin, when knowledge can be obtained. Parents should read and inform themselves in regard to the laws God has established in our beings. Instead of trying to allay with MEDICINE every trifling complaint, they might trace the disturbance to some defect in their nursing, or a change made in their food, air, clothing, or exercise, and they would be rewarded for their investigation, by soon seeing a change for the better.

"Parents should give their children abundance of fresh air. If they have kept them smothered with flannels, with windows and doors closed, fearing they would get their death of cold, let them make haste and reform, if they would save their children. You have not given the body any chance to breathe through the millions of little mouths which nature has provided for it; and in consequence, these pores have become clogged, and cannot perform the task allotted them, and so the internal organs have a double task thrown upon them, and the whole system is deranged. But now the doctor must be sent for, and if the little patients live through the terrible ordeal he prescribes, the credit is given to his skill, when the only reason they lived was, because they had a stronger hold on life than most such small members of the human family have."

1866—*The Health Reformer*, October 1, 1866.

"No woman should become a mother unless she is capable of being physician to her offspring. How can mothers turn over their tender children to the care of a strange physician, for him to dose them with DRUGS, the true nature of which she has no knowledge. Such a course is a sin in the sight of Heaven. Ignorance is no excuse for parents. Why do not those who take such responsibilities, educate themselves? They should read and investigate with a prayerful heart, until they can understand the wants of their children, and watch with jealous care, lest these little sunbeams, which are given them to lighten their pathway, be shrouded in darkness by disease and death. No stranger's hand should be trusted to perform those services for her dear ones, which a mother's affection alone can understand. Parents and children should educate themselves in all that concerns their life and health. When children understand the science of human life, then, and not till then, are they prepared to attend to the sciences as taught in the common schools.

"Parents have frequently told me that they knew nothing of the nature of disease, and were their children sick, they should not know what to do for them—that they had always trusted to a physician. Mothers ought to know what to do in any common case of sickness of their children. It is a sin for them not to know. Who should better understand the wants of a sick child than its parents, especially the mother? And yet parents plead ignorance, and if their dear children are slightly indisposed, they do not know what to do, and send for the doctor, who deals out his CONCENTRATED POISONS with a lavish hand. These lessen the child's hold on life, and if they do not actually cause its death, they obstruct nature's efforts, and break down some part of her fine machinery, which can never be repaired, and the victim is a sufferer as long as life lasts.

"In nine cases out of ten, the indisposition of children can be traced to some indulgence of the perverted appetites. Perhaps it is an exposure to cold, want of fresh air, irregularity in eating, or improper clothing; and all the parents need do, is to remove the cause, and secure for their children a period of quiet and rest, and abstain for a short period from food. An agreeable bath, of a proper temperature, will remove impurities from the skin, and then unpleasant symptoms may soon disappear; and all of this, too, without POISONOUS DRUGS, or having a doctor's fee to pay.

"Many parents, rather than to take the trouble to thoroughly investigate the cause of their children's indisposition, turn them over to the doctor, and administer anything he may choose to prescribe. If the anxious parent ventures to make an inquiry in regard to the DRUG, she is told it is 'perfectly harmless;' that if it does them no special good, 'it will not injure them.' CONCENTRATED POISONS are dealt out, the names of which are concealed in some technical terms, which the parents know nothing of; and because of their inexcusable ignorance, the lives of their children are sacrificed, and the parents too frequently charge their afflictions to Providence.

"In such cases perhaps, if nature had been left to herself, she would have recovered the abuse the system had suffered, but she was not allowed the privilege. A POISONOUS DRUG is introduced into the system, binding down the efforts of nature, until she is compelled to give up the struggle. Do the parents then see their folly, and awake and investigate for themselves, feeling that their children are too dear to be trusted in a stranger's hands to receive ANY MIXTURE he may please to deal out? No, they seem blinded, and infatuated; habits and customs, like iron bands, gird them about, and they make no effort to break them. If other loved ones are made sick by the wrong course pursued toward them, the doctor is again sent for to deal out his miserable DRUGS, which have so long cursed the human family and filled our graveyards, and the little life forces left, are crushed out, and death closes the scene.

"I have known instances where two or three in the same family have died, one after another, and yet the same physician was summoned to attend them all. I had not a doubt but that careful nursing, letting alone DRUGS entirely, with a little moral courage and firmness, used by the parents to restrict the diet of their children, would have saved them. There never can be a better condition of things, until parents understand the obligations resting upon them to bring up their children healthfully. It is impossible to conform to the present customs of society and do this. There is need of reform. Parents should live more for their children, and not so much for visitors. It should not be their study how to furnish a luxurious table to please the appetites of visitors. By so doing, they tempt their children to eat things which will prove injurious to health, and which will encourage and strengthen the animal appetites, and have a direct influence to weaken and debase the higher faculties.

"Children, judging of the course pursued by their parents, take it for granted that the highest object in life, and that which yields the greatest amount of happiness, is to be able to prepare a table spread with luxurious food. They are taught that we 'live to eat,' instead of 'eating to live.' The time devoted in studying how to prepare food in a manner to suit the perverted appetite, is worse than lost. Such knowledge is a curse to parents and children; for they are only learning the most successful way to tear down and debase the physical, mental, and moral faculties, by gluttony. Then, as a natural result, comes sickness, and next the doctor and POISONOUS DRUGS.

"It is thus that the human family are successfully destroying themselves, and deteriorating the race, and then they lay the result of their sinful course to a 'mysterious Providence.' Time, strength and money, are devoted to the unworthy object of keeping pace with fashionable customs of society, and the health of the body and soul is sacrificed to this end. Yet those who are guilty in this respect, will tell you they do not understand how to take care of themselves or their children, when sick. How much better would it be for parents and children, if the time and means that are devoted to preparing food to suit the depraved appetite, were occupied in acquiring a knowledge of their physical being, and in learning how to take care of their own bodies, and in teaching their children the same. Children should be taught, by precept and example, that God did not design that we should live merely for present gratification, but for our ultimate good. God has formed laws which govern our constitutions, and these laws which he has placed in

Spirit of Prophecy References

our being, are divine, and for every transgression there is affixed a penalty, which must sooner or later be realized. The majority of diseases which the human family have been, and still are suffering under, they have created by ignorance of their own organic laws. They seem indifferent in regard to the matter of health, and work perseveringly to tear themselves to pieces, and when broken down, and debilitated in body and mind send for the doctor and DRUG themselves to death."
(LP—*Counsels on Diet and Foods*, 19)

1867—*Review and Herald*, October 8, 1867.

"It was at the house of Brother A. Hilliard, at Otsego, Michigan, June 6, 1863, that the great subject of Health Reform was opened before me in vision. I did not visit Dansville till August, 1864, fourteen months after I had the view. I did not read any works upon health until I had written *Spiritual Gifts*, vols. 3 and 4, *Appeal to Mothers*, and had sketched out most of my six articles in the six numbers of *How to Live*. I did not know that such a paper existed as the *Laws of Life*, published at Dansville, New York. I had not heard of the several works upon health, written by Dr. J. C. Jackson, and other publications at Dansville, at the time I had the view named above. I did not know that such works existed until September, 1868, when in Boston, Massachusetts, my husband saw them advertised in a periodical called the *Voice of the Prophets*, published by Elder J. V. Himes. My husband ordered the works from Dansville and received them at Topsham, Maine. His business gave him no time to peruse them, and as I determined not to read them until I had written out my views; the books remained in their wrappers. As I introduced the subject of health to friends where I labored in Michigan, New England, and in the State of New York, and spoke against DRUGS and flesh meats, and in favor of water, pure air, and a proper diet, the reply was often made, 'You speak very nearly the opinions taught in the *Laws of Life*, and other publications, by Drs. Trall, Jackson, and others. Have you read that paper and those works?' My reply was that I had not, neither should I read them till I had fully written out my views, lest it should be said that I had received my light upon the subject of health from physicians, and not from the Lord. And after I had written my six articles for *How to Live*, I then searched the various works on hygiene and was surprised to find them so nearly in harmony with what the Lord had revealed to me. And to show this harmony, and to set before my brethren and sisters the subject as brought out by able

writers, I determined to publish *How to Live*, in which I largely extracted from the works referred to.
(*Selected Messages,* book 3, 277)

1867—*The Ellen G. White Biography*, 1862–1876, vol. 2, 76—Arthur L. White.

"Six months after the health reform vision, Henry, their oldest son, took sick with pneumonia, as already noted, and eight days later died. Why? Neither James White nor Ellen had yet had an opportunity to acquaint themselves with steps to take in combating disease through the use of rational methods. Some weeks before, James had sent for Dr. Jackson's books, but at the onset of Henry's severe illness the books were still in their wrappers (*Review and Herald*, October 8, 1867). They had been traveling and had had little time to read. Although the experienced physician had administered DRUGS, their son died. What a jolt this gave them. They doubtless recalled successfully treating diphtheria ten months earlier through the rational use of water and the application of other simple remedies."

1867—*Testimonies*, vol. 1, 502.

"The consciousness of right-doing is the best MEDICINE for diseased bodies and minds. The special blessing of God resting upon the receiver is health and strength. A person whose mind is quiet and satisfied in God is in the pathway to health. To have a consciousness that the eyes of the Lord are upon us and His ears open to our prayers is a satisfaction indeed. To know that we have a never-failing Friend in whom we can confide all the secrets of the soul is a privilege which words can never express. Those whose moral faculties are beclouded by disease are not the ones to rightly represent the Christian life or the beauties of holiness. They are too often in the fire of fanaticism or the water of cold indifference or stolid gloom. The Words of Christ are of more worth than the opinions of all the physicians in the universe: 'Seek ye first the kingdom of God, and his righteousness; and all these things shall be added unto you.' Matthew 6:33. This is the first great object—the kingdom of heaven, the righteousness of Christ. Other objects to be attained should be secondary to these."
(*Christian Temperance and Bible Hygiene*, 162; *The Health Reformer*, March 1, 1872; *Review and Herald*, March 12, 1872 and March 30, 1886)

1868—*Review and Herald*, March 24, 1868—James White and Ellen G. White

"In answer to many inquiries, we would say that we believe there is business for Seventh-day Adventists to enter upon for a livelihood, more consistent with their faith than the raising of HOPS, TOBACCO, or swine. (*Selected Messages*, book 2, 338)

"And we would recommend that they plant no more HOPS, or TO-BACCO fields, and that they reduce the number of their swine. They may yet see it duty, as most consistent believers do, to keep no more. We would not urge this opinion upon any. Much less would we take the responsibility of saying, 'Plow up your HOP and TOBACCO fields, and sacrifice your swine to the dogs.' (*Selected Messages*, book 2, 338)

"While we would say to those who are disposed to crowd HOP, TOBACCO, and swine growers among our people, that they have no right to make these things, in any sense, a test of Christian fellowship, we would also say to those who have these miserable things on hand, If you can get them off your hands without great loss, consistency with the faith of this people whose publications and oral teachings have so much to say on the subject of reform, more than suggests that you should get them off your hands as soon as possible." (*Selected Messages*, book 2, 338)

1868—*Review and Herald*, April 14, 1868.

"If those ladies who are failing in health, suffering in consequence of these diseases, would lay off their fashionable robes, clothe themselves suitably for the enjoyment of such exercise, and move out carefully at first, as they can endure it, and increase the amount of exercise in the open air as it gives them strength to endure, and dismiss their doctors and DRUGS, most of them might recover health, to bless the world with their example and the work of their hands. If they would dress their daughters properly, they might live to enjoy health, and to bless others." (*The Health Reformer*, September 1, 1868 and May 1, 1872; *Pamphlet 134, The Dress Reform*, 10)

1868—*Testimonies*, vol. 1, 695.

"Love can no more exist without revealing itself in outward acts than fire can be kept alive without fuel. You, Brother C, have felt that it was beneath your dignity to manifest tenderness by kindly acts, and to watch for an opportunity to evince affection for your wife by words of tenderness and kind regard. You are changeable in your feelings, and are very much affected by surrounding circumstances. You have not felt that it was wrong, displeasing to God, to allow your mind to be fully engrossed with the world, and then bring your worldly perplexities into

your family, thus letting the adversary into your home. It is very easy for you thus to open the door, but you will find it not so easy to close; it will be very difficult to turn out the enemy when once you have brought him in. Leave your business cares and perplexities and annoyances when you leave your business. Come to your family with a cheerful countenance, with sympathy, tenderness, and love. This will be better than expending money for MEDICINES or physicians for your wife. It will be health to the body and strength to the soul. Your lives have been very wretched. You have both acted a part in making them so. God is not pleased with your misery; you have brought it upon yourselves by want of self-control."
(F & LP—*The Adventist Home*, 111)

1868—*Testimonies*, vol. 2, 18.

"We returned home from this tour just before a great fall of rain which carried off the snow. This storm prevented the next Sabbath meeting, and I immediately commenced to prepare matter for *Testimony* No. 14. We also had the privilege of caring for our dear Brother King, whom we brought to our home with a terrible injury upon the head and face. We took him to our house to die, for we could not think it possible for one with the skull so terribly broken in to recover. But with the blessing of God upon a very gentle use of water, a very spare diet till the danger of fever was past, and well-ventilated rooms day and night, in three weeks he was able to return to his home and attend to his farming interests. He did not take one grain of MEDICINE from first to last. Although he was considerably reduced by loss of blood from his wounds and by spare diet, yet when he could take a more liberal amount of food he came up rapidly."
(*Life Sketches of Ellen G. White*, 185–186)

1868—*Testimonies*, vol. 2, 184–185.

"Sister T loves this world. She is naturally selfish. She has suffered much with bodily infirmities. God permitted this affliction to come upon her, and yet would not permit Satan to take her life. God designed through the furnace of affliction to loosen her grasp upon earthly treasures. Through suffering alone could this be done. She is one of those whose systems have been poisoned by DRUGS. By taking these she has ignorantly made herself what she is; yet God did not suffer her life to be taken, but lengthened her years of probation and suffering that she might become sanctified through the truth, be purified, made white and tried,

and, through the furnace of affliction, lose her dross, and become more precious than fine gold, even than the golden wedge of Ophir. Love of the {185} world has become so deeply rooted in the hearts of this brother and sister that it will require a severe trial to remove it. Dear brother and sister, you lack devotion to God. You are insane in regard to worldly things. The world has power to conform your mind to it, while the spiritual and heavenly do not bear with sufficient weight to transform the mind."
(*The Retirement Years,* 82)

1869—*An Appeal to Mothers,* 17–18.

"The state of our world was presented before me, and my attention was especially called to the youth of our time. Everywhere I looked, I saw imbecility, dwarfed forms, crippled limbs, misshapen heads, and deformity of every description. Sins and crimes, and the violation of nature's laws, were shown me as the causes of this accumulation of human woe and suffering. I saw such degradation and vile practices, such defiance of God, and I heard such words of blasphemy, that my soul sickened. From what was shown me, a large share of the youth now living are worthless. Corrupt habits are wasting their energies, and bringing upon them loathsome and complicated diseases. Unsuspecting parents will try the skill of one physician after another, who prescribe DRUGS, when they generally know the real cause of the failing health, but for fear of offending and losing their fees, they keep silent, when as faithful physicians they should expose the real cause. Their DRUGS only add a second great burden for abused nature to struggle against, which often breaks down in her efforts and the victim {18} dies. And the friends look upon the death as a mysterious dispensation of Providence, when the most mysterious part of the matter is, that nature bore up as long as she did against her violated laws. Health, reason, and life, were sacrificed to depraved lusts."

1870—*Testimonies,* vol. 2, 390–391.

"The Lord has given me a view of some of the corruptions everywhere existing. Wickedness, crime, and sensuality exist even in high places. Even in the churches professing to keep God's commandments there are sinners and hypocrites. It is sin, not trial and suffering, which separates God from His people and renders the soul incapable of enjoying and glorifying {391} Him. It is sin that is destroying souls. Sin and vice exist in Sabbathkeeping families. Moral pollution has done more than every other evil to cause the race to degenerate. It is practiced to an alarming extent and brings on disease of almost every description. Even very small children, infants, being born with natural irritability of the sexual organs, find momentary relief in handling them, which only increases the irritation, and leads to a repetition of the act, until a habit is established which increases with their growth. These children, generally puny and dwarfed, are prescribed for by physicians and DRUGGED; but the evil is not removed. The cause still exists."

(FP—*Pamphlet 85, Special Testimony for the Battle Creek Church,* 1–2; LP–*Healthful Living,* 216–217)

1870—*Testimonies,* vol. 2, 529.

"When the weather will permit, all who can possibly do so ought to walk in the open air everyday, summer and winter. But the clothing should be suitable for the exercise, and the feet should be well pro-tected. A walk, even in winter, would be more beneficial to the health than all the MEDICINE the doctors may prescribe. For those who can walk, walking is preferable to riding. The muscles and veins are enabled better to perform their work. There will be increased vitality, which is so necessary to health. The lungs will have needful action, for it is impos-sible to go out in the bracing air of a winter's morning without inflating the lungs."

(*Counsels on Health,* 52; *Healthful Living,* 130)

1871—*The Health Reformer,* March 1, 1871.

"We have not now the bracing air of winter to stimulate the system. Many will feel a sense of languor. They will feel indisposed to exercise, or to engage in labor which requires exertion, especially if their employment has been sedentary. Such need the vitalizing, out-of-door air. This will be a more safe and successful tonic than ANY DRUG that physicians may prescribe."

1871—*The Health Reformer,* June 1, 1871.

"Live, dear invalid friends, while you do live, and train yourselves to shed fragrance like the fresh flowers. If you are burdened and weary, you need not curl up like leaves upon a withered branch. Cheerfulness and a clear conscience are better than DRUGS, and will be an effective agent in your restoration to health. In order for you to be cheerful, you should have exercise. You should have something useful to do. Invalid sisters should have something to call them out of doors, to work in the ground. This was the employment given by God to our first parents. God

knew that employment was necessary to happiness. You should have a spot of ground to claim as yours, to tend and cultivate. You may have a pride in keeping out every weed, and may watch with interest the beautiful development of every leaf and opening bud and flower, and be charmed with the miracles of God seen in nature. As you view the shrubs and flowers, remember God loves the beautiful in nature. As you watch the harmonious colors of the various beautiful-tinted flowers of June, bear in mind that God loves the beautiful in human nature formed in His image. A pure, harmonious character, a sunny temper, reflecting light and cheerfulness, glorifies God, and benefits humanity. Inspiration tells us that a meek and quiet spirit in the sight of God is of great price."
(MP—*Mind, Character, and Personality,* vol.1, 322; *My Life Today,* 177; *Healthful Living,* 233)

1871—*The Health Reformer,* July 1, 1871.

"The truth is, the masses are led on blindly by popular physicians, who are the last men to engage in the work of informing the people. Their stronghold is in the superstitious confidence of the people, in their doses. Should they teach the people how to live so as to keep well, their practice would be ruined. But we rejoice to witness indications that many are awaking to the glad thought that it is their privilege to learn how to live so as to keep out of the doctor's hand, and that the pure air, pure water, quiet, abstinence from DRUGS, and a proper diet, are the best means that can be employed for the recovery of those who suffer from failing health."

1871—*The Health Reformer,* September 1871, —Mary H. Heald, M. D. as quoted by Ellen G. White.

"Let a person be habituated to the use of OPIUM, and upon ceasing to take the DRUG, he suffers intensely. The same with TOBACCO, ALCOHOL, COFFEE, TEA, flesh food, salt, and so on, and so on. But let one accustomed to a hygienic dietary cease to use one or more of the articles to which he is habituated, and he does not experience suffering from their disuse. There is no surer test of the amount of injury received by the system from the use of a STIMULANT or NARCOTIC than the measure of suffering occasioned by discontinuing the the use of the same."

1871—*The Health Reformer,* December 1, 1871.

"The heathen devotees sacrifice their lives to their gods. The car of Juggernaut crushes out the lives of many, and missionaries are sent to enlighten this benighted race. But why are not Christians aroused in our land

of boasted light and Christianity, as they witness the daily sacrifice of health and life among women to follow slavish customs that actually destroy a greater number of lives than are sacrificed among the heathen, and this in a land where Christ is preached? And what is worse, professing Christians take the lead, and set the example. How many who minister in the sacred desk, in Christ's stead, and are beseeching men to be reconciled to God, and are exalting the free gospel, who are themselves slaves to appetite, and are defiled with TOBACCO. They are daily weakening their nerve-brain power by the use of a filthy NARCOTIC. And these men profess to be ambassadors for the Holy Jesus. And thousands of Christians are destroying their vitality by becoming fashionable slaves in point of dress. Fashion will not give them room to breathe, or freedom of motion, and they submit to the torture. They lay aside reason and noble independence, and submit to the martyrdom of fashion, sacrificing health, beauty, and even life itself."
(MP—*Temperance,* 69)

1872—*Testimonies,* vol. 3, 21.

"Above all things, we should not with our pens advocate positions that we do not put to a practical test in our own families, upon our own tables. This is dissimulation, a species of hypocrisy. In Michigan we can get along better without salt, sugar, and milk than can many who are situated in the Far West or in the Far East, where there is a scarcity of fruit. But there are very few families in Battle Creek who do not use these articles upon their tables. We know that a free use of these things is positively injurious to health, and, in many cases, we think that if they were not used at all, a much better state of health would be enjoyed. But at present our burden is not upon these things. The people are so far behind that we see it is all they can bear to have us draw the line upon their injurious indulgences and STIMULATING NARCOTICS. We bear positive testimony against TOBACCO, SPIRITUOUS LIQUORS, SNUFF, TEA, COFFEE, flesh meats, butter, spices, rich cakes, mince pies, a large amount of salt, and all exciting substances used as articles of food."
(*Counsels on Diet and Foods,* 468; *Testimony Studies on Diet and Foods,* 11, 104, 130, 135, 148; *Pamphlet 159, Testimony to the Church,* 44–45)

1872—*Testimonies,* vol. 3, 172–173.

"The religion of the Bible is not detrimental to the health of the body or of the mind. The influence of the Spirit of God is the VERY BEST MEDICINE that can be received by a sick man or woman. Heaven is all health, and the more deeply the heavenly influences are realized the more sure will be the recovery of the believing invalid. At some other health institutions they encourage amusements, plays, and dancing to get up an excitement, but are fearful as to the result of a religious interest. Dr. Jackson's theory in this respect is not only erroneous but dangerous. Yet he has talked this in such a manner that, were his instructions heeded, patients would be led to think that their recovery depended upon their having as few thoughts of God and heaven as possible. It is true that there are persons with ill-balanced minds who imagine themselves to be very religious and who impose upon themselves fasting and prayer {173} to the injury of their health. These souls suffer themselves to be deceived. God has not required this of them. They have a pharisaical righteousness, which springs, not from Christ, but from themselves. They trust to their own good works for salvation and are seeking to buy heaven by meritorious works of their own instead of relying, as every sinner should, alone upon the merits of a crucified and risen Saviour. Christ and true godliness, today and forever, will be health to the body and strength to the soul."

(FP—*The Health Reformer*, October 1, 1872)

1873—*The Health Reformer*, June 1, 1873.

"I have observed a great deficiency in so-called educated ladies. They may have graduated with honors, but are shamefully deficient in the practical duties of life. They are destitute of the qualifications necessary for the proper regulation and happiness of the family. They may talk of woman's elevated sphere and of her rights, while they themselves sink far below the true sphere of woman. God designed that women should become intelligent in the most essential duties of life. But very many in the scale of knowledge and efficiency are even below their hired servants. It is the right of every daughter of Eve in our land to be thoroughly educated in household duties, having a knowledge of all the branches of practical life in domestic labor. She may preside in her family as queen in her domain, her household being her kingdom. She should be fully competent to direct her servants. It is woman's right to be qualified to direct the expanding minds of her children. It is her right to have an understanding of her own and her children's organisms, that she may know how to treat her children, and save them from the POISONS of doctors' DRUGS. She may adore her gracious Creator as she contemplates how beautifully and simply nature carries on her work when she is not interfered with. She may be an intelligent nurse and physician of her own dear children, instead of leaving their precious lives in the hands of stranger physicians, to be DRUGGED to death. It is woman's right to know how to regulate her own habits, and those of her children, in diet and dress, in exercise and in domestic duties, and employment in the open air in relation to life and health."

1874—*Review and Herald,* September 8, 1874.

"It is impossible for these to realize the binding claims and holiness of the law of God. The brain and nerves are deadened by the use of this NARCOTIC. They cannot value the atonement or appreciate the worth of immortal life. The indulgence of fleshly lusts wars against the soul. The apostle in the most impressive manner addresses Christians, 'I beseech you therefore, brethren, by the mercies of God, that ye present your bodies a living sacrifice, holy, acceptable unto God.' Romans 12:1. If the body is saturated with LIQUOR and the defilement of TOBACCO, it is not holy and acceptable to God. Satan knows that it cannot be, and for this reason he brings his temptations to bear upon men upon the point of appetite, that he may bring them into bondage to this propensity and thus work their ruin."

(Redemption; or the Temptation of Christ In the Wilderness, 61; The Health Reformer, March 1, 1878)

1875—*Review and Herald,* March 25, 1875.

"Notwithstanding they have this striking example before them, some professed Christians will desecrate the house of God with breaths polluted with the fumes of LIQUOR and TOBACCO. And the spittoons are sometimes filled with the ejected spittle and quids of TOBACCO. The effluvia is constantly arising from these receptacles, polluting the atmosphere. Men professing to be Christians bow to worship God, and dare to pray to Him with their lips stained by TOBACCO, while their half-paralyzed nerves tremble from the exhausting use of this POWERFUL NARCOTIC. And this is the devotion they offer to a holy, and sin-hating God. Ministers in the sacred desk, with mouth and lips defiled, dare to take the sacred Word of God in their polluted lips. They think God does not notice their sinful indulgence. 'Because sentence against an evil work is not executed speedily, therefore the heart of the sons of men is fully set in them to do evil.' Ecclesiastes 8:11. God will no more receive a sacrifice from the hands of those who thus pollute themselves, and offer with their service the incense of TOBACCO and LIQUOR, than he

would receive the offering of the sons of Aaron, who offered incense with strange fire."
(Redemption: or the Temptation of Christ In the Wilderness, 85–86)

1875—*Review and Herald,* July 22, 1875.

"It was under very discouraging circumstances that Elder Bourdeau presented the truth to them. The opposition from prejudiced minds was very bitter. But some honest souls were interested, and when brought up to face the mirror, to compare their lives with the law of God, they were deeply convicted of sin. One brother who is now rejoicing in the truth, and can say with Paul, 'I was alive without the law once: but when the commandment came, sin revived, and I died,' (Romans 7:9) when he came to view his life in the light of the holy law, saw his sins to be so exceedingly sinful, that he thought they were too great to be forgiven. He was in great agony of mind. He called together his neighbors and friends, and confessed to them the sins and wrongs of his life, and entreated their forgiveness. He tried to right every wrong. This wonderful work of the power of God in convicting the sinner, was a thing so new to his friends and neighbors that they thought he was out of his mind, and feared that he would die. Several physicians were consulted, and MEDICINE was prescribed freely. But DRUGS, which would be useless to cure the diseased body, were utterly powerless to cure the sin-sick soul. While suffering the most intense remorse of conscience for his sins, the Lord did not leave him to perish. The light of health reform was forced upon his mind, and he refused to take the DRUGS prescribed, for he was strongly convinced that they were POISON, and ruinous to his constitution."

1875—*Testimonies,* vol. 3, 488.

"The only safe course is to touch not, taste not, handle not, TEA, COFFEE, WINES, TOBACCO, OPIUM, and ALCOHOLIC DRINKS. The necessity for the men of this generation to call to their aid the power of the will, strengthened by the grace of God, in order to withstand the temptations of Satan and resist the least indulgence of perverted appetite is twice as great as it was several generations ago. But the present generation have less power of self-control than had those who lived then. Those who have indulged the appetite for these STIMULANTS have transmitted their depraved appetites and passions to their children, and greater moral power is required to resist intemperance in all its forms. The only perfectly safe course to pursue is to stand firmly on the side of temper-

ance and not venture in the path of danger."
*Counsels on Health, 125; The Health Reformer, August 1, 1875.
FP—Counsels on Diet and Foods, 428; Temperance, 163; Healthful Living, 112;
Testimony Studies on Diet and Foods, 147)*

1875—*Testimonies*, vol. 3, 561, 567–569.

"Those who have been overcome on the point of appetite and are using TOBACCO freely are debasing their mental and moral powers and bringing them into servitude to the animal. And when the appetite for SPIRITUOUS LIQUOR is indulged, the man voluntarily places to his lips the draft which debases below the level of the brute him who was made in the image of God. Reason is paralyzed, the intellect is benumbed, the animal passions are excited, and then follow crimes of the most debasing character. If men would become temperate in all things, if they would touch not, taste not, handle not, SPIRITUOUS LIQUORS and NARCOTICS, reason would hold the reigns of government in her hands and control the animal appetites and passions. In this fast age the less exciting the food the better. Temperance in all things and firm denial of appetite is the only path of safety. . . .{567}

"Parents may have transmitted to their children tendencies to appetite and passion, which will make more difficult the work of educating and training these children to be strictly temperate and to have pure and virtuous habits. If the appetite for unhealthy food and for STIMULANTS and NARCOTICS has been transmitted to them as a legacy from their parents, {568} what a fearfully solemn responsibility rests upon the parents to counteract the evil tendencies which they have given to their children! How earnestly and diligently should the parents work to do their duty, in faith and hope, to their unfortunate offspring! . . .
(Child Guidance, 405; Counsels on Health, 609; Mind, Character, and Personality, vol. 1, 140; Temperance, 174–175; Testimony Studies on Diet and Foods, 60–61; Counsels on Diet and Foods, 236–237; FP—Counsels for the Church, 103)

"Satan is corrupting minds and destroying souls through his subtle temptations. Will our people see and feel the sin of indulging perverted appetite? Will they discard TEA, COFFEE, flesh meats, and all stimulating food, and devote the means expended for these hurtful indulgences to spreading the truth? These STIMULANTS do only harm, and yet we see that a large number of those who profess to be Christians are using TOBACCO. These very men will deplore the evil of intemperance, and while speaking against the use of LIQUORS will eject the juice of TOBACCO. While a healthy state of mind depends upon the normal condition of the vital forces, what care should be exercised that neither STIMU-

LANTS nor NARCOTICS be used."
(Counsels on Health, 85; Testimony Studies on Diet and Foods, 164)

1876—*The Signs of the Times*, January 6, 1876.

"Gluttonous feasting and the indulgence of NARCOTICS and STIMULANTS, are carried to great lengths even by the Christian world. How many close their last precious hours of probationary time, in scenes of gaiety, feasting and amusement, where serious thoughts are not allowed to enter, where the spirit of Jesus would be unwelcome! Their last precious hours are passing while their minds are benumbed with TOBACCO and ALCOHOLIC LIQUORS. There are not a few who pass directly from the dens of infamy to the sleep of death; they close their life-record among the associations of dissipation and vice. What will the awakening be at the resurrection of the unjust! . . .

"Those who profess to be the followers of Christ yet have this terrible sin at their door, cannot have a high appreciation of the atonement and an elevated estimate of eternal things. Minds that are clouded and partially paralyzed by NARCOTICS, are easily overcome by temptation, and cannot enjoy communion with God."
(Temperance, 64; LP—To Be Like Jesus, 313)

1876—*Testimonies*, vol. 4, 32.

"It is not an easy matter to overcome an established taste for NARCOTICS and STIMULANTS. In the name of Christ alone can this great victory be gained. He overcame in behalf of man in the long fast of nearly six weeks in the wilderness of temptation. He sympathizes with the weakness of man. His love for fallen man was so great that He made an infinite sacrifice that He might reach him in his degradation and through His divine power finally elevate him to His throne. But it rests with man whether Christ shall accomplish for him that which He is fully able to do."

1877—*The Health Reformer*, January 1, 1877.

"I would appeal to parents to devote less time to ornamenting their children's clothing, which only fosters in them a spirit of vanity, and to so instruct them that they may secure good constitutions. And then they can dismiss doctors with their DRUGS, and see their children enjoy good health, sound morals, and standing independent for a sensible, healthful dress in defiance of the fashions of our times."

Spirit of Prophecy References

1877—*The Health Reformer*, September 1, 1877.

"God forbid that woman should degrade herself to the use of a filthy and besotting NARCOTIC. How disgusting is the picture which one may draw in the mind, of a woman whose breath is poisoned by TOBACCO. One shudders to think of little children twining their arms about her neck, and pressing their fresh, pure lips to that mother's lips, stained and polluted by the offensive fluid and odor of TOBACCO. Yet the picture is only more revolting because the reality is more rare than that of the father, the lord of the household, defiling himself with the disgusting weed. No wonder we see children turn from the kiss of the father whom they love, and if they kiss him seek not his lips, but his cheek or forehead, where their pure lips will not be contaminated."

(*Temperance*, 59; *The Signs of the Times*, December 6, 1877)

1878—*The Signs of the Times*, January 3, 1878.

"Many now are convicted, and God's Spirit is striving with them, but they will not heed the invitations of mercy. Men who make high profession of wisdom and of godliness transgress the law of God without compunctions of conscience. One marked feature of Noah's day was the intense worldliness of the inhabitants. They were eating and drinking, planting and building, marrying and giving in marriage, not that these things were of themselves sins, but they were, although lawful in themselves, carried to a high degree of intemperance. The appetite was indulged at the expense of health and reason. This constant indulgence of their sinful desires corrupted them and defiled the earth under them. The same evils intensified exist in our world today. Men are blind to reason and the result of indulging perverted appetite. The world is the god of nine-tenths of professed Christians. The indulgence of appetite is carried to the greatest excess. TOBACCO, WINE, LIQUOR and OPIUM are added to the list of a feverish stimulating diet."

1878—*The Health Reformer*, July 1, 1878.

"When ministers, from their pulpits, make loyalty to the law of God disreputable; when they join with the world in making it unpopular; when these teachers of the people indulge in the social glass, and the defiling NARCOTIC, TOBACCO—what depth of vice may not be expected from the youth of this generation? The newspaper records of the day, with their annals of crime, murders, and suicides, give the answer, and point out the terrible dangers of the time. . . .

Spirit of Prophecy References

"The Christian church is pronounced to be the salt of the earth, the light of the world. Can we apply this to the churches of today, many of whose members are using, not only the defiling NARCOTIC, TOBACCO, but INTOXICATING WINE, and SPIRITUOUS LIQUOR, and are placing the WINE-CUP to their neighbor's lips? The church of Christ should be a school in which the inexperienced youth should be educated to control their appetites, from a moral and religious standpoint. They should there be taught how unsafe it is to tamper with temptation, to dally with sin; that there is no such thing as being a moderate and temperate drinker; that the path of the tippler is ever downward. They should be exhorted to 'look not upon the WINE when it is red,' which 'at the last biteth like a serpent, and stingeth like an adder.' Proverbs 23:31–32."

(*The Signs of the Times*, August 29, 1878; *Temperance*, 164–165)

1878—*The Health Reformer*, October 1, 1878.

"It is not an easy matter to overcome established habits of taste and appetite for NARCOTICS and STIMULANTS. In the name of Christ alone can this great victory be gained. He overcame in behalf of man in the wilderness of temptation, in the long fast of nearly six weeks. He sympathizes with the weakness of fallen man. His love for him was so great that He made an infinite sacrifice that He might reach him in his degradation, and through His divine power elevate him finally to His throne. But it rests with man whether Christ shall accomplish for him that which He has undertaken and is fully able to do."

1878—*The Signs of the Times*, October 31, 1878.

"It is not an easy matter to overcome established habits of appetite for NARCOTICS and STIMULANTS. In the name of Christ alone can this great victory be gained. He overcame in behalf of man in the wilderness of temptation, in the long fast of nearly six weeks. He sympathizes with the weakness of fallen man. His love for him was so great that He made an infinite sacrifice that He might reach him in his degradation, and through His divine power elevate him finally to His throne. But it rests with man whether Christ shall accomplish for him that which He has undertaken and is fully able to do."

1879—*Testimonies*, vol. 4, 309.

"These words of Christ should sink into the hearts of all who believe present truth: 'And take heed to yourselves, lest at any time your hearts be overcharged with surfeiting, and drunkenness, and cares of this life, and so that day come upon you unawares.' Luke 21:34. Our danger is presented before us by Christ Himself. He knew the perils we should meet in these last days, and would have us prepare for them. 'As it was in the days of Noe, so shall it be also in the days of the Son of man.' Luke 17:26. They were eating and drinking, planting and building, marrying and giving in marriage, and knew not until the day that Noah entered into the ark, and the Flood came and swept them all away. The day of God will find men absorbed in like manner in the business and pleasures of the world, in feasting and gluttony, and in indulging perverted appetite in the defiling use of LIQUOR and the NARCOTIC TOBACCO. This is already the condition of our world, and these indulgences are found even among God's professed people, some of whom are following the customs and partaking of the sins of the world. Lawyers, mechanics, farmers, traders, and even ministers from the pulpit are crying, 'Peace and safety,' when destruction is fast coming upon them. 1 Thessalonians 5:3."

(*Review and Herald,* October 20, 1885 and August 16, 1887; *Testimony Studies on Diet and Foods,* 164; *The Signs of the Times,* October 8, 1902)

1880—*Review and Herald,* March 11, 1880.

"The consciousness of right-doing is the best MEDICINE for diseased bodies and minds. The special blessing of God is health and strength to the receiver. A person whose mind is quiet and satisfied in God is in the pathway to health. To have a consciousness that the eyes of the Lord are upon us, and his ears open to hear our prayers, is a satisfaction indeed. To know that we have a never-failing Friend in whom we can confide all the secrets of the soul, is a privilege which words can never express. The Words of Christ are of more worth than the opinions of all the physicians in the universe. 'Seek ye first the kingdom of God, and his righteousness; and all these things shall be added unto you.' Matthew 6:33. This is the first great object—the kingdom of Heaven, the righteousness of Christ. The attainment of all other objects should be secondary to this."

1880—*The Signs of the Times,* July 1, 1880.

"This is the purpose of Satan, to belittle the requirements of God, and make of none effect His Holy Law. The man of sin has placed a common working day in the very bosom of the Decalogue and in doing this has thought to change the law of God and has thus exalted himself above God. Were the moral powers of man clear and vigorous they would not choose the common in the place of the sacred because it is more convenient to be in harmony with the world. The general disobedience of man does not change or detract one particle from the positive command to keep holy the seventh day, for God placed His sanctity upon that day. A principle of right and obedience to God are always and everywhere the only safe rule. The language of every God-fearing soul should be, Perish whatever may, gold, silver, houses, lands, reputation, but let me retain my integrity and the approval of God. The habit of doing wrong in breaking one of God's commandments will not lessen the guilt. There are habits contracted by bad example, or by bad influence before we have judgment to discern the right; or the force of reason may be so narcotized by indulgence of appetite in the use of TOBACCO, OPIUM and LIQUOR that wrong is not discerned. These slaves to appetite are completely under the dominion of their master, and unless evil habits are conquered, they will conquer and destroy."

1880—*The Signs of the Times*, July 8, 1880.

"Men who make laws to control the people should above all others be obedient to the higher laws which are the foundation of all rule in nations and in families. How important that men who have a controlling power should themselves feel they are under a higher control. They will never feel thus while their minds are weakened by indulgence in NARCOTICS, and STRONG DRINK. Those to whom it is intrusted to make and execute laws should have all their powers in vigorous action. They may, by practicing temperance in all things, preserve the clear discrimination between the sacred and common, and have wisdom to deal with that justice and integrity which God enjoined upon ancient Israel. Man may cultivate his powers, and with invincible determination rise to the high standard God has set for him in His Word. Then with wisdom he may judge uprightly and with a sense that the eye of God is upon him, he will not swerve from the right, but will be kind, sympathizing, despising bribes, and governed by the highest motives in all his service.
(*Temperance*, 46–47)

"Many who are elevated to the highest positions of trust in serving the public are the opposite of this. They are self-serving, and generally indulge in the use of NARCOTICS, and WINE and STRONG DRINK. Lawyers, jurors, senators, judges, and representative men have forgotten that they cannot dream themselves into a character. They are deterio-

rating their powers through sinful indulgences. They stoop from their high position to defile themselves with intemperance, licentiousness, and every form of evil. Their powers prostituted by vice opens their path for every evil. An elevated position of trust does not make the man after God's own heart, but too frequently it leads him to despise persevering labor, and to forget that sin alone will make man really mean and low. He who toils in earnest labor, striving to make the most of his God-given powers, in homage and love to his Creator is doing his work as faithfully in his sphere as are the cherubim and seraphim in their most sacred work, and loftiest ministrations.
(FP—*Temperance,* 47)

"Intemperate men should not by vote of the people be placed in positions of trust. Their influence corrupts others, and grave responsibilities are involved. With brain and nerve narcotized by TOBACCO and stimulus they make a law of their nature, and when the immediate influence is gone there is a collapse. Frequently human life is hanging in the balance; on the decision of men in these positions of trust, depends life and liberty, or bondage and despair. How necessary that all who take part in these transactions should be men proved, men of self-culture, men of honesty and truth, of staunch integrity, who will spurn a bribe, who will not allow their judgment or convictions of right to be swerved by partiality or prejudice. Thus saith the Lord, 'Thou shalt not wrest the judgment of thy poor in his cause. Keep thee far from a false matter; and the innocent and righteous slay them not: for I will not justify the wicked. And thou shalt take no gift: for the gift blindeth the wise, and perverteth the words of the righteous.' Exodus 23:6–8.
(*Temperance,* 47; *To Be Like Jesus,* 177)

"In order to carry out these stern principles of right, intemperance is positively forbidden of God. God requires that the faculties of man should be well-balanced, the judgment clear and discriminating, that ideas may be received through the senses and compared with one another, investigating calmly, patiently, critically, evidences presented and arranging the matter with the action of sound judgment without a faculty being perverted. This was God's purpose, and He forbids on penalty of death that the gifts of intellect He has bestowed upon man shall be subverted by NARCOTICS or stimulus of any kind, that the talents He has intrusted to man may be a tower of strength to the people, in the place of a power to ruin and destroy. All who would meet the mind of God and come off conquerors, must bid adieu to ease, luxury, flattery, and vice, and arm

Spirit of Prophecy References

themselves for the mighty, soul-testing struggle against indulgence of appetite."

1881—*Review and Herald*, January 25, 1881.

" 'Abstain from fleshly lusts, which war against the soul,' (1 Peter 2:11) is the language of the apostle Peter. Many regard this warning as applicable only to the licentious; but it has a broader meaning. It guards against every injurious gratification of appetite or passion. It is a most forcible warning against the use of such STIMULANTS and NARCOTICS as TEA, COFFEE, TOBACCO, ALCOHOL, and MORPHINE. These indulgences may well be classed among the lusts that exert a pernicious influence upon moral character. The earlier these hurtful habits are formed, the more firmly will they hold their victim in slavery to lust, and the more certainly will they lower the standard of spirituality. . . .
(*Counsels on Diet and Foods*, 62–63; *Counsels on Health*, 67–68; *Temperance*, 73; *Testimony Studies on Diet and Foods*, 27)

"Those who are in the habit of using TEA, COFFEE, TOBACCO, OPIUM, or SPIRITUOUS LIQUORS, cannot worship God when they are deprived of the accustomed indulgence. Let them, while deprived of these STIMULANTS, engage in the worship of God, and divine grace would be powerless to animate, enliven, or spiritualize their prayers or their testimonies. These professed Christians should consider the means of their enjoyment. Is it from above, or from beneath?"
(Counsels on Diet and Foods, *426;* Testimony Studies on Diet and Foods, *147)*

1881—*The Signs of the Times*, September 22, 1881.

"The effect of STIMULANTS and NARCOTICS is to lessen physical strength; and whatever affects the body, will affect the mind. A STIMULANT may for a time arouse the energies and produce mental and physical activity; but when the exhilarating influence is gone, both mind and body will be in a worse condition than before. Intoxicating LIQUORS and TOBACCO have proved a terrible curse to our race, not only weakening the body and confusing the mind, but debasing the morals. As the control of reason is set aside, the animal passions will bear sway. The more freely these POISONS are used, the more brutish will become the nature and disposition of men."
(*Bible Echo and Signs of the Times*, March 1, 1887.
FP—*Child Guidance*, 404)

1881—*Manuscript Releases*, vol. 2, 107.

"TEA, COFFEE, TOBACCO, and ALCOHOL we must present as sinful indulgences. We cannot place on the same ground, meat, eggs, butter, cheese and such articles placed upon the table. These are not to be borne in front, as the burden of our work. The former—TEA, COFFEE, TOBACCO, BEER, WINE, and all SPIRITUOUS LIQUORS—are not to be taken moderately, but discarded. The POISONOUS NARCOTICS are not to be treated in the same way as the subject of eggs, butter, and cheese. In the beginning animal food was not designed to be the diet of man. We have every evidence that the flesh of dead animals is dangerous because of disease that is fast becoming universal, because of the curse resting more heavily in consequence of the habits and crimes of man. We are to present the truth. We are to be guarded how to use reason and select those articles of food that will make the very best blood and keep the blood in an unfevered condition."

(*Selected Messages,* book 3, 287–288; *Review and Herald,* June 25, 1959)

1881—*Review and Herald,* November 8, 1881.

"Many men are voted into office whose minds are deprived of their full vigor by indulgence in SPIRITUOUS LIQUORS, or constantly beclouded by the use of the NARCOTIC TOBACCO. How often have the decisions made by courts of justice fastened suspicion upon those whose characters were untainted, wrenched hard-earned means from the rightful owners, or perchance immured innocent men in prison cells. And all this because the mental and moral powers of judge, jurors, or witnesses, mayhap [perhaps] of all, were impaired by the use of NARCOTICS or STIMULANTS. Who can feel secure when so many whose duty it is to enact or execute the laws, pervert judgment under the influence of these POISONS? The peace of happy families, reputation, property, liberty, and even life itself, are at the mercy of intemperate men in our legislative halls and our courts of justice."

(LP—*Temperance,* 254)

1882—*The Signs of the Times,* February 2, 1882.

"I could but think of the large sums paid annually in doctors' bills, or in the purchase of HURTFUL or POISONOUS DRUGS. If the means thus often worse than wasted could be spent in visiting such a resort as is afforded in this delightful place, how many might be benefited physically and mentally. Our people should purchase this establishment, and make of it a Hygienic Institute, as was the original intention of its founders. New buildings ought to be erected, and all needed facilities added to make it in all respects a first-class institution. It should be opened in the spring for the reception of patients."

Spirit of Prophecy References

1882—*The Signs of the Times*, March 2, 1882.

"Let old and young remember that for every violation of the laws of life, nature will utter her protest. The penalty will fall upon the mental as well as the physical powers. And it does not end with the guilty trifler. The effects of his misdemeanors are seen in his offspring, and thus hereditary evils are passed down, even to the third or fourth generation. Think of this, fathers, when indulging in the soul-and-brain-benumbing NARCOTIC, TOBACCO. Where will this practice leave you? Whom will it affect besides yourself? . . .

"OPIUM, TEA, COFFEE, INTOXICATING LIQUORS, and TOBACCO are extinguishing as fast as they well can, the spark of vitality left for the race. We are suffering for the wrong habits of our fathers, and yet how many take a course in every way worse than they. Can any be called Christians who thus willfully destroy themselves?"

1882—*Review and Herald*, May 16, 1882.

"In a health institution we provide a place where the sick can enjoy the benefit of nature's remedial agents, instead of depending upon DEADLY DRUGS. And many who thus find relief, will be ready to yield to the influence of the truth."

1882—*Selected Messages*, book 2, 302–303.

"I have not knowingly drunk a cup of genuine COFFEE for twenty years, only, as I stated, during my sickness—for a MEDICINE—I drank a cup of {303} COFFEE, very strong, with a raw egg broken into it."

1882—*Testimonies*, vol. 5, 194–195.

"Many are unwilling to put forth the needed effort to obtain a knowledge of the laws of life and the simple means to be employed for the restoration of health. They do not place themselves in right relation to life. When sickness is the result of their transgression of natural law, they do not seek to correct their errors and then ask the blessing of God, but they resort to the physicians. If they recover health they give to DRUGS and doctors all the honor. They are ever ready to idolize human power and wisdom, seeming to know no other God than the creature—dust and ashes. . . .

(*Counsels on Health*, 45; *Christian Temperance and Bible Hygiene*, 112; *Review and Herald*, June 27, 1882)

Spirit of Prophecy References

"Go with me to yonder sickroom. There lies a husband and father, a man who is a blessing to society and to the cause of God. He has been suddenly stricken down by disease. The fire of fever seems consuming him. He longs for pure water to moisten the parched lips, to quench the raging thirst, and cool the fevered brow. But, no; the doctor has forbidden water. The stimulus of STRONG DRINK is given and adds fuel to the fire. The blessed, heaven-sent water, skillfully applied, would quench the devouring flame; but it is set aside for POISONOUS DRUGS."
(*Review and Herald,* June 27, 1882;
LP—*Healthful Living,* 214)

1882—*The Signs of the Times,* June 15, 1882.

"The consciousness of right-doing, is the best MEDICINE for diseased bodies and minds. He who is at peace with God has secured the most important requisite to health. The blessing of the Lord is life to the receiver. The assurance that the eye of the Lord is upon us, and his ear open to our prayer, is a never-failing source of satisfaction. To know that we have an all-wise friend, to whom we can confide all the secrets of the soul, is a privilege which words can never express."
(*Healthful Living,* 233)

1882—*Good Health,* November 1, 1882.

"Peter's admonition to abstain from fleshly lusts (see 1 Peter 2:11) is a most direct and forcible warning against the use of all such STIMULANTS and NARCOTICS as TEA, COFFEE, TOBACCO, ALCOHOL, and MORPHINE. These indulgences may well be classed among the lusts that exert a pernicious influence upon moral character. . . ."
(*The Sanctified Life,* 28)

"When those who are in the habit of using TEA, COFFEE, TOBACCO, OPIUM, or SPIRITUOUS LIQUORS, are deprived of the accustomed indulgence, they find it impossible to engage with interest and zeal in the worship of God. Divine grace seems powerless to enlighten or spiritualize their prayers or their testimonies. These professed Christians should consider the source of their enjoyment. Is it from above, or from beneath?"
(*Temperance,* 74; *The Sanctified Life,* 32)

1882—*Review and Herald,* November 21, 1882.

"It is not an easy matter to overcome established habits, to deny the appetite for NARCOTICS and STIMULANTS. In the name of Christ alone can this great victory be gained. Our Saviour paid a dear price for man's redemption. In the wilderness of temptation He suffered the

keenest pangs of hunger; and while emaciated with fasting, Satan was at hand with his manifold temptations to assail the Son of God, to take advantage of His weakness and overcome Him, and thus thwart the plan of salvation. But Christ was steadfast. He overcame in behalf of the race, that He might rescue them from the degradation of the fall. Christ's experience is for our benefit. His example in overcoming appetite points out the way for those who would be His followers, and finally sit with Him on His throne. The Son of God sympathizes with the weaknesses of man. His love for the fallen race was so great that He made an infinite sacrifice to reach man in his degradation, and through His divine power elevate him finally to His throne. But it rests with man whether Christ shall accomplish for him that which He is fully able to do."
(*Good Health,* March 1, 1883)

1882—*Review and Herald,* December 26, 1882.

"Many Sabbathkeepers neglect to take the *Review,* and some have neither the *Review* nor the *Signs.* They plead as an excuse that they cannot afford to take these papers which it is so important for them to have. But in many cases several secular papers will be found upon their tables for their children to peruse. The influence of most of the periodicals of the day is such as to render the Word of God distasteful, and to destroy a relish for all useful and instructive reading. The mind assimilates to that which it feeds upon. The secular papers are filled with accounts of murders, robberies and other revolting crimes, and the mind of the reader dwells on the scenes of vice therein depicted. But indulgence, the reading of sensational or demoralizing literature becomes a habit, like the use of OPIUM or other BALEFUL DRUGS, and as a result, the minds of thousands are enfeebled, debased, and even crazed. Satan is doing more through the productions of the press to weaken the minds and corrupt the morals of the youth than by any other means."
(*The Publishing Ministry,* 376; *Counsels to Writers and Editors,* 133–134)

1884—*Review and Herald,* January 29, 1884.

"At Denver we were told that we must go into a smoking-car, and at the same time no restriction was placed upon the smokers. When one or two were asked to forego smoking, they decidedly refused, declaring they should smoke all they chose to, and neither men nor women should hinder them. If any did not like it, 'let them keep out of the car.' These men were TOBACCO SLAVES. They had lost their sense of manly politeness, and did not care for their appearance. If they would abandon the use of the disgusting, defiling NARCOTIC, and then could see its effects on the physical, mental, and moral powers, they would exclaim, as we felt like saying, 'The Lord deliver us from such associates, and from such degrading bondage!' "

1884—*Review and Herald,* March 25, 1884.

"I have received letters from different individuals, inquiring if I think it in accordance with our faith to raise HOPS, knowing that they are principally used in the manufacture of INTOXICATING DRINKS, or to engage in the manufacture of WINE or CIDER for the market."

"I cannot see how, in the light of the law of God, Christians can conscientiously engage in these pursuits. All these articles may be put to a good use, and prove a blessing; and they may be perverted to a wrong use, and prove a temptation and a curse."

1884—*The Signs of the Times,* May 1, 1884.

"The consciousness of right-doing is the best MEDICINE for diseased bodies and minds. The special blessing of God resting upon the receiver is health and strength. Those whose moral faculties are clouded by disease are not the ones to rightly represent the Christian life or the beauties of holiness. They are too often in the fire of fanaticism, or the water of cold indifference or stolid gloom. The Words of Christ are of more worth than the opinions of all the physicians in the universe: 'Seek ye first the kingdom of God, and his righteousness; and all these things shall be added unto you.' Matthew 6:33. This is the first great object—the kingdom of Heaven, the righteousness of Christ. Other objects to be attained should be secondary." (*Mind, Character, and Personality,* vol.1, 34)

1884—*Counsels on Diet and Foods,* 406.

"The Health Retreat was established at a great cost to treat the sick without DRUGS. It should be conducted on hygienic principles. DRUG MEDICATION should be worked away from as fast as possible, until entirely discarded. Education should be given on proper diet, dress, and exercise. Not only should our own people be educated, but those who have not received the light upon health reform should be taught how to live healthfully, according to God's order. But if we have no standard in this respect ourselves, what is the need of going to such large expense to establish a health institute? Where does the reform come in?" (*Testimony Studies on Diet and Foods,* 111)

1884—*Manuscript Releases,* vol. 19, 284.

"The smoking steamboat inspector was told it was the TOBACCO smoke which had acted like POISON upon me. He threw away his CIGAR and we had no more smoking on the train. A physician on board stated that he feared it was to me a fatal POISON and that I would never become conscious again. He told me never to consent to be in the room or in the car, carriage, or steamboats where I would be obliged to breathe the air poisoned by TOBACCO, for he had in his practice treated many cases of mothers and children with affection of the heart caused by living in and inhaling constantly TOBACCO-POISONED AIR. Notwithstanding he warned the husband and father of the sure result, he thought there could have been no change [in the man's habit], for the afflicted ones lived only a short time and were [as] verily poisoned to death as if a dose of ARSENIC or STRYCHNINE had been administered. The blood was poisoned."

1884—*Manuscript Releases,* vol. 19, 343.

"It was through intemperate appetite that Adam and Eve lost Eden, and it will be through habits of strict temperance and denial of hurtful indulgences that we shall have calm nerves and mental acuteness to discern good from evil. A man who is intemperate, who uses stimulating indulgences—BEER, WINE, STRONG DRINKS, TEA and COFFEE, OPIUM, TOBACCO, or any of these substances that are deleterious to health—cannot be a patient man. So temperance is a round of the ladder upon which we must plant our feet before we can add the grace of patience. In food, in raiment, in work, in regular hours, in healthful exercise, we must be regulated by the knowledge which it is our duty to obtain, that we may through earnest endeavor place ourselves in right relation to life and health."
(*Our High Calling,* 69)

1884—*Review and Herald,* July 29, 1884.

"Our ancestors have bequeathed to us customs and appetites which are filling the world with disease. The sins of the parents, through perverted appetite, are with fearful power visited upon the children to the third and fourth generations. The bad eating of many generations, the gluttonous and self-indulgent habits of the people, are filling our poorhouses, our prisons, and our insane asylums. Intemperance in drinking TEA and COFFEE, WINE, BEER, RUM, and BRANDY, and the use of TOBACCO, OPIUM, and other NARCOTICS, has resulted in great mental and physical degeneracy, and this degeneracy is constantly increasing."

(Counsels on Health, 49; Mind, Character, and Personality, vol.1, 144; Temperance, 174)

1884—*Selected Messages,* book 2, 283.

"Do not administer DRUGS. True, DRUGS may not be as dangerous wisely administered as they usually are, but in the hands of many they will be hurtful to the Lord's property."

1884—*The Signs of the Times,* October 23, 1884.

"The consciousness of right-doing is the best MEDICINE for diseased bodies and minds. The special blessing of God resting upon the receiver, is health and strength. One whose mind is quiet and satisfied in God is on the highway to health. To have the consciousness that the eye of the Lord is upon us, and that his ear is open to our prayers, is a satisfaction indeed. To know that we have a never-failing Friend to whom we can confide all the secrets of the soul, is a happiness which words can never express. Those whose moral faculties are clouded by disease are not the ones to rightly represent the Christian life or the beauties of holiness. They are too often in the fire of fanaticism, or the water of cold indifference or stolid gloom."

(Reflecting Christ, 161; Counsels on Health, 628)

1885—*Review and Herald,* February 10, 1885.

"The work of this institution, as indicated in the various reports of the superintendent, is largely that of personal instruction to each patient upon the causes that lead to alcoholism, the effect upon the physical system and upon the mental and moral character, and the means to be used in overcoming the habit, and in antidoting this POISON which has been imbibed into the system, and which permeates the whole being of man. The system of reform is not MEDICINAL; it is not a system of DRUGGING and purging, nor a gradual tapering off in the use of ALCOHOL. The watchword at the portals of this institution is total abstinence from ALCOHOL in every form. There are no ALCOHOLIC TINCTURES in MEDICINES, no mild tonics, reinforced by other STIMULANTS or NARCOTICS, but total abstinence from the use of ALCOHOL in any form, whether mixed with malt, QUININE, ginger, eggs, milk, CIDER, or lemonade."

1885—*Mind, Character, and Personality,* vol. 2, 691.

"There are some who use NARCOTICS, and by indulgence are encouraging wrong habits that are obtaining a controlling power over the will, the thoughts, and the entire man."

Spirit of Prophecy References

1885—*Testimonies*, vol. 5, 311.

"My dear friends, instead of taking a course to baffle disease, you are petting it and yielding to its power. You should avoid the use of DRUGS and carefully observe the laws of health. If you regard your life you should eat plain food, prepared in the simplest manner, and take more physical exercise. Each member of the family needs the benefits of health reform. But DRUGGING should be forever abandoned; for while it does not cure any malady, it enfeebles the system, making it more susceptible to disease."

(*Counsels on Diet and Foods*, 82–83;
LP—*Healthful Living*, 65, 244)

1885—*Testimonies*, vol. 5, 356, 358–359.

"I cannot see how, in the light of the law of God, Christians can conscientiously engage in the raising of HOPS or in the manufacture of WINE or CIDER for the market. All these articles may be put to a good use and prove a blessing, or they may be put to a wrong use and prove a temptation and a curse. CIDER and WINE may be canned when fresh and kept sweet a long time, and if used in an unfermented state they will not dethrone reason. But those who manufacture apples into CIDER for the market are not careful as to the condition of the fruit used, and in many cases the juice of decayed apples is expressed. Those who would not think of using the poisonous, rotten apples in any other way will drink the CIDER made from them and call it a luxury; but the microscope would reveal the fact that this pleasant beverage is often unfit for the human stomach, even when fresh from the press. If it is boiled, and care is taken to remove the impurities, it is less objectionable. . . . {358}

(FP—*Counsels on Diet and Foods*, 432–433; *Testimony Studies on Diet and Foods*, 14.)

"When intelligent men and women who are professedly Christians plead that there is no harm in making WINE or CIDER for the market because when unfermented it will not intoxicate, I feel sad at heart. I know there is another side to this subject that they refuse to look upon; for selfishness has closed their eyes to the terrible evils that may result from the use of these STIMULANTS. I do not see how our brethren can abstain from all appearance of evil and engage largely in the business {359} of HOP RAISING, knowing to what use the HOPS are put. Those who help to produce these beverages that encourage and educate the appetite for STRONGER STIMULANTS will be rewarded as their works

have been. They are transgressors of the law of God, and they will be punished for the sins which they commit and for those which they have influenced others to commit through the temptations which they have placed in their way."
(*Temperance,* 98; *Review and Herald,* March 25, 1904)

1885—*Testimonies,* vol. 5, 439–443.

"The physician should be a strictly temperate man. The physical ailments of humanity are numberless, and he has to {440} deal with disease in all its varied forms. He knows that much of the suffering he seeks to relieve is the result of intemperance and other forms of selfish indulgence. He is called to attend young men, and men in the prime of life and in mature age, who have brought disease upon themselves by the use of the NARCOTIC TOBACCO. If he is an intelligent physician he will be able to trace disease to its cause, but unless he is free from the use of TOBACCO himself he will hesitate to put his finger upon the plague spot and faithfully unfold to his patients the cause of their sickness. He will fail to urge upon the young the necessity of overcoming the habit before it becomes fixed. If he uses THE WEED himself, how can he present to the inexperienced youth its injurious effects, not only upon themselves, but upon those around them?"
(*Counsels on Health,* 321–322)

"In this age of the world the use of TOBACCO is almost universal. Women and children suffer from having to breathe the atmosphere that has been polluted by the PIPE, the CIGAR, or the foul breath of the TO-BACCO USER. Those who live in this atmosphere will always be ailing, and the smoking physician is always prescribing some DRUG to cure ailments which could be best remedied by throwing away TOBACCO.

"Physicians cannot perform their duties with fidelity to God or to their fellow men while they are worshiping an idol in the form of TO-BACCO. How offensive to the sick is the breath of the TOBACCO USER! How they shrink from him! How inconsistent for men who have gradu-ated from medical colleges and claim to be capable of ministering to suffering humanity, to constantly carry a POISONOUS NARCOTIC with them into the sickrooms of their patients. And yet many chew and smoke until the blood is corrupted and the nervous system undermined. It is especially offensive in the sight of God for physicians who are capable of doing great good, and who profess to believe the truth of God for this time, to indulge in this disgusting habit. The words of the apostle Paul are applicable to them: 'Having therefore these promises, dearly beloved, let us cleanse ourselves from all filthiness of the flesh and spirit, {441} perfecting holiness in the fear of God.' 2 Corinthians 7:1. 'I beseech you therefore, brethren, by the mercies of God, that ye present your bodies a living sacrifice, holy, acceptable unto God, which is your reasonable service.' Romans 12:1. . . . {442}

"Our Saviour set an example of self-denial. In His prayer for His disciples He said: 'For their sakes I sanctify myself, that they also might be sanctified through the truth.' John 17:19. If a man who assumes so grave a responsibility as that of a physician sins against himself in not conforming to nature's laws, he will reap the consequences of his own doings and abide her righteous decision, from which there can be no appeal. The cause produces the effect; and in many cases the physician, who should have a clear, sharp mind and steady nerves, that he may be able to discern quickly and execute with precision, has disordered nerves and a brain clouded by NARCOTICS. His capabilities for doing good are lessened. He will lead others in the path his own feet are traveling. Hundreds will follow the example of one intemperate physician, feeling that they are safe in doing what the doctor does. And in the day of God he will meet the record of his course and be called to give an account for all the good he might have done, but did not do because by his own voluntary act he weakened his physical and mental powers by selfish indulgence. . . . {443}

"There are many ways of practicing the healing art, but there is only one way that Heaven approves. God's remedies are the simple agencies of nature that will not tax or debilitate the system through their powerful properties. Pure air and water, cleanliness, a proper diet, purity of life, and a firm trust in God are remedies for the want of which thousands are dying; yet these remedies are going out of date because their skillful use requires work that the people do not appreciate. Fresh air, exercise, pure water, and clean, sweet premises are within the reach of all with but little expense, but DRUGS are expensive, both in the outlay of means and in the effect produced upon the system. . . .
(*Counsels on Diet and Foods,* 301; *Counsels on Health,* 323; *Pamphlet 49, Loma Linda's Work,* 1)

"The physician should know how to pray. In many cases he must increase suffering in order to save life; and whether the patient is a Christian or not, he feels greater security if he knows that his physician fears God. Prayer will give the sick an abiding confidence; and many

times if their cases are borne to the Great Physician in humble trust, it will do more for them than all the DRUGS that can be administered."
(*Counsels on Health*, 324)

1886—*The Signs of the Times*, February 11, 1886.

"Let old and young remember that for every violation of the laws of life, nature will utter her protest. The penalty will fall upon the mental as well as the physical powers. And it does not end with the guilty trifler. The effects of his misdemeanors are seen in his offspring, and thus hereditary evils are passed down, even to the third or fourth generation. Think of this, fathers, when you indulge in the use of the soul-and-brain-benumbing NARCOTIC, TOBACCO. Where will this practice leave you? Whom will it affect besides yourselves? . . .
(*Temperance*, 56)

"We are suffering for the wrong habits of our fathers, and yet how many take a course every way worse than theirs! Every year millions of gallons of INTOXICATING LIQUORS are drank, and millions of dollars are spent for TOBACCO. OPIUM, TEA, COFFEE, TOBACCO, and INTOXICAT-ING LIQUORS are rapidly extinguishing the spark of vitality still left in the race. And the slaves of appetite, while constantly spending their earn-ings in sensual indulgence, rob their children of food and clothing and the advantages of education."
(*Reflecting Christ*, 142)

1887—*Review and Herald*, April 19, 1887.

"Jesus endured the painful fast in our behalf, and conquered Satan in every temptation, thus making it possible for man to conquer in his own behalf, and on his own account, through the strength brought to him by this mighty victory gained as man's Substitute and Surety. We thank the Lord that a victory was gained upon these points, even here in Basel; and we hope to carry our brethren and sisters up to a still higher standard to sign the pledge to abstain from JAVA COFFEE and the HERB that comes from China. We see that there are some who need to take this step in reform. There are some who are nervous, and they should abstain from these nerve-weakening NARCOTICS, that they may place themselves in right relation to the laws of life and health. These INJURI-OUS STIMULANTS are doing great harm to their nervous system. The machinery of nature is aroused to unwonted activity to be followed by reaction, and the COFFEE and TEA must be used by them to keep up their strength and again urge up their powers. Unnatural activity is the result, and by this continual course of indulgence of appetite the natural vigor of the constitution becomes gradually and imperceptibly impaired. If we would preserve a healthy action of all the powers of the system, nature must not be forced to unnatural action. Nature will stand at her post of duty, and do her work wisely and efficiently, if the false props that have been brought in to take the place of nature are expelled. (FP—*Ellen G. White in Europe 1885-1887*, 271)

1887—*Counsels on Health*, 441.

"We thank the Lord that a victory has been gained, but we hope to carry our brethren and sisters up to a still higher standard, where they will sign the pledge to abstain from COFFEE and the HERB that comes from China."

1887—*Manuscript Releases*, vol. 5, 24.

"Mary has been an apprentice in this office, but has not been well for some time. The blood is mostly in her head. Sara McEnterfer has been treating her for months—fomentations, foot baths, sponge baths, rubbings, and so on. A physician was called to give her an examination. He says her case is a complicated one, and she must leave the office. Her parents were afraid to have her come home, because I had set before them the poisonous atmosphere in the house, which they were inhaling all the time. I saw that the precious child would not get well here, so I finally proposed that Mary should go to America, to the sanitarium. They consented to let her go. Now I wish you to tell me if this is not the best thing to be done. The physicians here do not know how to take a case without DRUGGING. They commended the way that she has been treated, and recommended her to go to an institution in Basel, under the care of the physician that attended Edith Andrews. The treatment is all given by men with masks on. Mary is a modest young woman, and she would not go there, she said, if she died. What do you think of my sending her to the sanitarium? She has had a hard time the past winter—her feet cold as ice, room not properly heated. Her ankles swell very badly. She came down unable to do anything. I could not spare Sara. She would work over her hours at a time, and I thought I would better be to the expense of her treatment at the sanitarium than have Sara take care of her here without conveniences whatever."

1887—*The Paulson Collection of Ellen G. White Letters*, 21–25.

"I have found it no easy matter to secure means to invest in health institutions. But it has proved a still more difficult matter to secure per-

sons who were qualified to conduct such institutions. It requires thoroughly balanced characters to do this work, not men who have some strong traits of character, but who are weak as children in other points. Plenty of physicians can be obtained who ceased to be students when they received their diplomas, who are self-inflated, who feel that they know all that is worth knowing, and what they do not know is not worth knowing. But this class are not the ones we want. When a physician enters upon his work as a practitioner, the more genuine, practical experience he has, the more fully will he feel his want of knowledge. If self-sufficient, he will read articles written in regard to disease and how to treat them without nature's aid; he will grasp statements and weave them into his practice, and without deep research, without earnest study, without sifting every statement, he will merely become a mechanical worker. Because he knows so little, he will be ready to experiment upon human lives, and sacrifice not a few. This is murder, actual murder. He did not do this work with evil design, he had no malicious purposes; but life was sacrificed on account of his ignorance, because he was a superficial student, because he had not had that practice that would make him a safe man to be entrusted with human lives. It requires care taking, deep, earnest taxation of the mind to carry the burden a physician should carry in learning his trade thoroughly. Every physician who has received a thorough education will be modest in his claims. It will not do for him to run any risk upon experimenting on human life, lest he be guilty of murder, and this be written against him in the books of heaven. There should be a careful, competent physician who will deal scarcely ever in DRUGS, and who will not boast that POWERFUL POISONS are far more effective than a smaller quantity carefully taken, It is true, it kills, if it does not cure; but DRUGS never cure. They change the order of difficulties, but never heal them, never remove the cause."
(*Manuscript Releases*, vol. 15, 274–275;
LP—*Medical Ministry*, 139–140)

"We have deeply regretted that there were not a large number of institutions working from the hygienic principles that are now in existence. All these cannot be prepared upon a large scale, involving large expense; but the question is, will they preserve the principles of hygiene, or will they use the easier method of using DRUGS, to take the place of treating diseases without resorting to DRUG MEDICATIONS? There could be many hygienic institutions in all parts of our world, if there were plenty of means and plenty of persons who had the qualifications to manage such institutions. The physicians who shall be employed should not only have a book knowledge, but a practical experience to understand disease and its causes, and will feel the necessity, as soon as they are brought into positions of trust, to commence the work of carrying the burden necessary for them to bear, in order to do the most careful, thorough work. They will, if they are not closely connected with God, become careless and venturesome. The first labors of a physician should be to educate the sick and suffering the very course they should {22} pursue to prevent disease. The greatest good can be done by our trying to enlighten the minds of all we can obtain access to, as to the best course for them to pursue to prevent sickness and suffering, and broken constitutions, and premature death; but those who do not care to undertake work that taxes their physical and mental powers will be ready to prescribe DRUG MEDICATION, which lays a foundation in the human organism for a twofold greater evil than that which they claim to have relieved.

(*Manuscript Releases*, vol. 15, 275–276; *Medical Ministry*, 221–222; *Selected Messages*, book 2, 282)

"A physician who has the moral courage to peril (imperil) his reputation in enlightening the understanding by plain facts, in showing the nature of disease and how to prevent it, and the dangerous practice of resorting to DRUGS, will have an uphill business, but he will live and let live. He will not use his POWERFUL DRUG MEDICATION, because of the knowledge he has acquired by studying books. He will, if a reformer, talk plainly in regard to the false appetites and ruinous self-indulgence, in dressing, in eating and drinking, in overtaxing to do a large amount of work in a given time, which has a ruinous influence upon the temper, the physical and mental powers. Knowledge is what is needed. DRUGS are too often promised to restore health, and the poor sick are so thoroughly DRUGGED with QUININE, MORPHINE, or some strong health-and life-destroying (word illegible), that nature may never make sufficient protest, but give up the struggle; and they may continue their wrong habits with hopeful impunity. Right and correct habits, intelligently and perseveringly practiced will be removing the cause of disease, and the STRONG DRUGS need not be resorted to. Many go on from step to step with their natural indulgences, which is bringing in just as unnatural condition of things as possible.

(*Manuscript Releases*, vol. 15, 276;
F & LP—*Medical Ministry*, 222;
FP—*Temperance*, 86–87; *Selected Messages*, book 2, 282–283;
LP—*Mind, Character, and Personality*, vol. 2, 597)

Spirit of Prophecy References

"Diseases of every stripe and type have been brought upon human beings by the use of TEA and COFFEE and the NARCOTICS, OPIUM and TOBACCO. These hurtful indulgences must be given up, not only one, but all; for all are hurtful, and ruinous to the physical, mental, and moral powers, and should be discontinued from a health standpoint. The common use of the flesh of dead animals has had a deteriorating influence upon the morals, as well as the physical constitution. Ill health in a variety of forms, if effect could be traced to the cause, would reveal the sure result of flesh eating. The disuse of meats, with healthful dishes nicely prepared to take the place of flesh meats, would place a large number of the sick and suffering ones in a fair way of recovering their health, without the use of DRUGS. But if the physicians encourage a meat-eating diet to his invalid patients, then he will make a necessity for the use of DRUGS. Nature will want some assistance to bring things to their proper condition, which may be found in the simplest remedies, especially in the use of nature's own furnished remedies—pure air, and with a precious knowledge of how to breathe; pure water, with a knowledge of how to apply it; plenty of sunlight in every room, if possible, in the house, and with an intelligent knowledge of what advantages are to be gained by its use. All these are powerful in their efficiency, and the patient who has obtained a knowledge of how to eat and dress healthfully, may live for comfort, for peace, for health; and will not be prevailed upon to put to his lips DRUGS, which, in the place of helping nature, paralyzes her powers. If the sick and suffering will do only as well as they know in regard to living out the principles of health reform perseveringly, they will, in nine cases out of ten, recover from their ailments.

(Manuscript Releases, vol. 15, 277–278;
FP—Medical Ministry, 222; Testimony Studies on Diet and Foods, 175; Counsels on Diet and Foods, 421;
LP—Medical Ministry, 223–224; Testimony Studies on Diet and Foods, 85)

"The feeble and suffering ones must be educated line upon line, precept {23} upon precept, here a little, and there a little, until they will have respect for, and live in obedience to, the law that God has made to control the human organism. Those who sin against knowledge and light, and resort to the skill of a physician in administering DRUGS, will be constantly losing their hold on life. The less there is of DRUG DOSING, the more favorable will be their recovery to health. DRUGS, in the place of helping nature, are constantly paralyzing her efforts. The health institutions for the sick will be the best places to educate the suffering ones to live in accordance with nature's laws and cease their health-destroying

practices in wrong habits in diet, in dress, that are in accordance with the world's habits and customs, which are not at all after God's order, they are doing a good work to enlighten our world.
(FP—*Manuscript Releases,* vol. 15, 278; *Medical Ministry,* 224)

"DRUGS always have a tendency to break down and destroy vital forces, and nature becomes so crippled in her efforts, that the invalid dies, not because he needed to die, but because nature was outraged. If she had been left alone, she would have put forth her highest efforts to save life and health. Nature wants none of such help as so many claim that they have given her. Lift off the burdens placed upon her, after the customs of the fashion of this age, and you will see in many cases nature will right herself. The use of DRUGS is not favorable or natural to the laws of life and health. The DRUG MEDICATION gives nature two burdens to bear, in the place of one. She has two serious difficulties to overcome, in the place of one. There is now positive need even with physicians, reformers in the line of treatment of disease, that greater painstaking effort be made to carry forward and upward the work for themselves, and to interestedly instruct those who look to them for medical skill to ascertain the cause of their infirmities. They should call their attention in a special manner to the laws which God has established, which cannot be violated with impunity. They dwell much on the working of disease, but do not, as a general rule, arouse the attention to the laws which must be sacredly and intelligently obeyed in such to prevent disease. Especially [is this true] if the physician has not been correct in his dietetic practices, if his own appetite has not been restricted to a plain, wholesome diet, in a large measure discarding the use of the flesh of dead animals, [if] he loves meat, [and] he has educated and cultivated a taste for unhealthful food. His ideas are narrow, and he will as soon educate and discipline the taste and appetite of his patients to love the things that he loves, as to give them the sound principles of health reform. He will prescribe for sick patients, flesh meats, when it is the very worst diet that they can have; it stimulates, but does not give strength. They do not inquire into their [patients'] former habits of eating and drinking, and take special notice of their erroneous habits which have been for many years laying the foundation of disease. Conscientious physicians should be prepared to enlighten those who are ignorant, and should with wisdom make out their PRESCRIPTIONS, prohibiting those things in their diet which he knows to be erroneous. He should plainly state the things which he regards as detrimental to the laws of health,

and leave these suffering ones to work conscientiously to do those things for themselves which they can do, and thus place themselves in the right relation to the laws of life and health. When from an enlightened conscience they do the very best they know how to do, to preserve themselves in health, then in faith they may look to the great Physician, who is a Healer of the body as well as of the soul. We are {24} health reformers. Physicians should have wisdom and experience, and be thorough health reformers. Then they will be constantly educating by precept and example their patients from DRUGS. For they well know that the use of DRUGS may produce for the time being favorable results, but which will implant in the system that which will cause great difficulties hereafter, which they may never recover from during their lifetime. Nature must have a chance to do her work. Obstructions must be removed, and opportunity given her to exert her healing forces, which she will surely do, if every abuse is removed from her, and she has a fair chance.
(*Manuscript Releases,* vol. 15, 278–280; *Medical Ministry,* 223–225)

"The sick should be educated to have confidence in nature's great blessings which God has provided, and the most effective remedies for disease are pure soft water; the blessed God-given sunshine coming into the rooms of the invalids; living outdoors as much as possible; having healthful exercise; eating and drinking in foods that are prepared in the most healthful manner. To resort to the DRUGGING process lays upon nature a most fearful, merciless burden from which they may never recover. There are many laboring under chronic diseases. They will swallow anything in the line of DRUGS prescribed by the unbelieving physician, when an intelligent knowledge that they are indulging in unnatural appetites which explains to them the cause of their suffering, if Christians, they would place themselves in a position as health reformers. They would change the cause which produces this sure result.
(*Testimony Studies on Diet and Foods,* 85; *Manuscript Releases,* vol. 15, 280–281.)

"There are many, many afflicted in our world with TOBACCO POISON, but the physicians who are summoned to treat their patients under painful afflictions brought upon them by TOBACCO USING—are not instructed by these worldly physicians to let the POISONS alone, in order that they may recover health; for many of these physicians use these POISONS themselves. How can they, then, consistently enlighten the understanding of those who indulge in the POISONOUS NARCOTIC, TOBACCO? The physician, if he is not a novice, can trace the effects back

to the true cause, but he dares not forbid its use, because he indulges in it himself. Some will in an undecided, halfway manner advise the TOBACCO USERS to take less of this NARCOTIC; but he does not say to them, This habit is killing you. They prescribe DRUGS to cure a disease which is the result of indulging unnatural appetites, and two evils are produced in the place of removing one.
(*Manuscript Releases,* vol. 15, 281;
F&LP—*Medical Ministry,* 225)

"Thousands need to be educated patiently, kindly, tenderly, but decidedly, that nine-tenths of their complaints are created by their own course of action. The more they introduce DRUGS into the system, the more certainly do they interfere with the laws of nature and bring about the very difficulties they DRUG themselves to avoid. Let everyone who contemplates erecting an institution, carefully consider whether they are to make it an institution conducted upon the principles of health reform, or whether they design to copy the popular institutions all through our land. If an institution for health is conducted upon the principles of health reform, it will require for its management a large amount of faith, large amount of patience, a large amount of perseverance, a large amount of moral power, such as they have scarcely dreamed of, to make such an institution a success and to pay its own way. The managers will require moral backbone, as well as superior educated skill. Lectures need to be given in such an institution everyday upon some points connected with the customs and habits of the people, of disease and its causes, and the only true course to be taken to prevent disease. All connected with our health institutions as managers and helpers should {25} possess the very best ability, should have abundance of Christian courtesy, should practice universally Christian politeness, should be tender, pitiful, courteous. This is positively essential in order to leave the right impression upon the minds of sick people. While trying to educate them away from the habits and customs of the world, many will be glad to be enlightened, while many who are wedded to their own fashionable, health-destroying indulgences will be offended, and make it very unpleasant for those who wish to do them good; and some have not the moral courage to keep right on in the fear of the Lord. There is even among those who have intelligence in regard to the laws of life and health, a constant selfish indulgence in those things which are injurious to both soul and body. There is intemperance in eating, and in the many varieties of food taken at one meal. In the preparation of food, there are unhealthful mixtures

which ferment in the stomach, and cause great distress. And yet these go on, continuing their indulgence, which lays the foundation for numerous difficulties. If these would have self-control, and educate their taste to eat only those things which the abused stomach can and will assimilate, they would save large expense in doctor bills, and avoid great sufferings."
(*Manuscript Releases,* vol. 15, 281–283

1888—*The Signs of the Times,* February 17, 1888.

"We want a work of reformation in our land. There are thousands who can testify to the benefits of discarding these luxuries, and drinking from nature's pure fountain. Why should we go to China and Japan for the products of a backward civilization? Why not banish the NARCOTIC BEAN and the POISONOUS HERB, and come into harmony with the sanitary laws of the Bible? If we are pursuing a course of action that brings weakness upon us, how can we present to God a holy offering, a living sacrifice? We are required to love God with all our hearts and our neighbor as ourselves; but we are failing of this high requirement, if we are unfitting ourselves by hurtful habits for rendering acceptable service to our Maker and to our fellow men. How can we think deeply and seriously on the plan of salvation, if our minds are clouded, our nerves unstrung, and our bodies full of pain and disease? If we are knowingly transgressing the laws of health, God cannot sustain and comfort us with His grace. This would only encourage us in wrong-doing. We must put our feet in the path of righteousness, and make all the efforts we can to walk uprightly, and then we may appropriate the rich promises, and we shall realize that we are kept by the power of God through faith unto salvation."

1888—*Healthful Living,* 247–248.

"Many physicians are not as thorough and intelligent as they should be in the practice of their profession. They resort to DRUGS, when greater skill and knowledge would teach them a more excellent way. Lives have been lost which might have been saved if DRUGS had not been resorted to. As a rule, the less frequently they are employed, the better the patient will prosper."
(FP—*Healthful Living,* 264)

"Make use of the remedies that God has provided. Pure air, sunshine, and the intelligent use of water are beneficial agents in the restoration of health. But the use of water is considered too laborious. It is

easier to employ DRUGS than to use natural remedies.
(*Temperance,* 85)

"In treating the sick, the physician will seek God for wisdom; then, instead of placing his dependence upon DRUGS and expecting that MEDI-CINE will bring health to his patients, he will use nature's {248} restoratives, and employ natural means whereby the sick may be aided to recover. The Lord will hear and answer the prayers of the Christian physician."

1888—*Manuscript Releases,* vol. 12, 379.

"Whatever course he may take he is only a man liable to make mistakes and give some a chance to find something to criticize. Because you do not always think and speak and act as one having the mind of Christ, you will not consider that you make mistakes and that others may criticize you. The position the doctor occupies in medical circles leads him amid scenes of temptation, where he needs a constant hold upon God and brethren who can help him, pray for him, advise and counsel him. If he has this hold he will be the means of great good. Some of the worldly wise will at first disapprove; lawless and designing ones, and those who are disaffected, and men who have apostatized from the faith, will plot against him, but if he maintains his integrity, as did Daniel, God will give him favor among men in order that true hygienic principles and appliances may prevail to a large extent over DRUG MEDICATION. Shall those who claim to be reformers cease to reform? Shall they set themselves in array against the work of reform and these men to whom the Lord shall entrust a certain work?"
(*The Ellen G. White 1888 Materials,* 101)

1888—*Manuscript Releases,* vol. 13, 371.

"Tell those who are sick that if the hosts of those who are dyspeptics and consumptives could turn farmers they might overcome disease, dispense with DRUGS and doctors, and recover health. But farmers themselves must get educated to give heed to the laws of life and health by regulating their labor, even if there is some loss in their grain or the harvesting of crops. Farmers work too hard and too constantly, and violate the laws of God in their physical nature. This is the worst kind of economy. For a day he may accomplish more, yet in the end he is a loser by his ill-management of himself."

1888—*Manuscript Releases,* vol. 18, 333.

"It is no denial of faith to use rational remedies judiciously. Water,

air, and sunshine, these are God's healing agents. The use of certain HERBS that the Lord has made to grow for the good of man, is in harmony with the exercise of faith."
(LP—*Pamphlet 144, The Place of Herbs in Rational Therapy*, 4)

1888—*Manuscript Releases*, vol. 20, 364.

"I had several conversations with Dr. Maxson and his wife. Their only reason for resigning, they stated, was the methods of treating in DRUG MEDICATION. Dr. Gibbs was, they said, a homeopathist; but this is not the case. He is an eclectic physician, and had, when he came to the Health Retreat, eight years of successful practice. Dr. Maxson and his wife stated that homeopathy was of the devil—it was like spiritism and mesmerism—and they could not conscientiously connect with him, although Dr. Gibbs, he acknowledged, had always treated him like a gentleman and had given him far greater liberty and freedom than he would have given Dr. Gibbs, were he in his place.

"I told Dr. Maxson we did not erect an institution at such immense cost to have people educated to resort to DRUGS, but to instruct them how to cure without DRUGS. I told them what the Lord had been pleased to show me nearly thirty years ago in regard to the old-school practice of DRUG MEDICATION upon the miserable wrecks of humanity, made so by the use of DRUGS. I told him of the two systems; the old-school system had killed thousands and its tens of thousands, while the eclectic, or, as he called it, homeopathy, had done no such deadly work. But this, I am sure, had no weight with him, for he frequently repeated the same thing. Finally he sent in his resignation. We tried to have him and his wife remain upon a different plan: we could form a training school, and Dr. Maxson and wife could educate in regard to hygienic principles and how to give treatment. But they declined to do this, and left."

1888—*Manuscript Releases*, vol. 20, 373–375.

"When the great question of health reform was opened before me, the methods of treating the sick were plainly revealed to me. The old-school, cruel practice and the sure results, where one claimed to be benefited, thousands were made lifelong invalids who, had they never seen a physician, would have recovered of themselves without implanting in their system diseases of a most distressing character. Eclectic was less dangerous. The homeopathy, which creates so deadly opposition from the regular practice, was attended with far less evil consequences than the old-school practice, but did much harm because it could be resorted to so easily and used so readily with so little expense. Many practice upon themselves and fall back upon this without real knowledge of their ailments, and do great harm to themselves. Proper regulation of their diet, abstinence from TEA, COFFEE, and all spices and flesh meats, gaining an intelligent knowledge of temperance, would be MEDICINE above all DRUGS.

"But Dr. Maxson has insisted in putting his manner of treatment in a false light. He has repeatedly stated that if Dr. Gibbs did not use DRUGS he was afloat and could not do anything. In Oakland I had another conversation with Dr. Maxson, and I urged him not to make so wonderful a specialty of methods of DRUG USING. I told him [that] after the whole system of DRUG MEDICATION had been laid open before me, I was shown of God that we should have an institution conducted on hygienic principles, {374} and in that institution lectures should be given not on how to use DRUGS, not to lead minds and educate them in the methods of DRUG USING, but to teach people the better way—to live healthfully and do without DRUGS. The words were repeated, Educate! Educate! Educate!

"I then saw that an intelligent knowledge of pure air, and use of it wisely and abundantly, and simple healthful food taken into the stomach temperately, eating and drinking to the glory of God, and ten thousand would be well who are now sick. Then I was taken from room to room and shown disease and its causes, and the result of DRUG MEDICATION. I was then shown through rooms of a hygienic institution that was conducted on hygienic principles and these simple means—sunlight, pure air, healthful habits. Constant instruction needs to be given, line upon line, precept upon precept, in regard to the necessity of clean bodies, clean houses, and clean premises. Breathing clean air would preserve health without the use of DRUGS.

"But to deny self, to restrict the appetite, to eat only wholesome food and exercise temperance in eating the wholesome food, abstaining almost wholly from the flesh of dead animals that creates nine-tenths of [the] disease in our world, is too severe a process for a large part of our world and of professed Christians to enter into; so they eat and drink without reference to health, and the result is a depraved condition of the system; then they resort to the [use of] DRUGS, because that is easiest, and there continues to be wicked disregard of the laws of life and of health in taking care to preserve good health. . . .

Spirit of Prophecy References

"The use of water to help the sick, plenty of exercise, education as to how to breathe, education as to purity of habits, would throw DRUGS in the shade in their own place, where they naturally belong. . . . {375}

"In Oakland I tried to show Dr. Maxson that his ideas were not after God's order in the set ideas that he could not harmonize with Dr. Gibbs. You say you have had an education in hygiene. Now, Dr. Maxson, you have all the opportunity in the world in the Rural Health Retreat to practice that education and demonstrate to Dr. Gibbs the fact that hygiene will do wonderful things. Just demonstrate this. Do not, if you see hard work in this practice like so many, leave it aside and resort to your STRONG DOSES of DRUGS. I have positive light that this is tampering with human life.

"But notwithstanding all I could say, he would go over the same ground again, presenting the infallibility of the allopathy above the home-opathy. I was sure all that I had said of the light which the Lord had been pleased to give me was in his mind as thistledown before the mind. He has asserted that he used less DRUGS than Dr. Gibbs, while Dr. Gibbs declares it is otherwise.

"But there has been positive harm done by the STRONG DOSES of MEDICINE given by Dr. Maxson—such enormous quantities of QUININE given to his patients, which he maintains is far better in influence than less. We have not a knowledge of the same results following the use of DRUGS from Dr. Gibbs. Dr. Maxson had things his own way for many weeks, for Dr. Gibbs was away. He had all the opportunity to lecture, all the room to work that he chose, and then Dr. Gibbs did not stand in his way at all—let him have all the room he asked.

1888—*Testimonies on Sexual Behavior, Adultery, and Divorce, 161–162.*

"In a dream on another occasion you were presented before me. Your head was bowed down upon a table. You were almost unconscious. Words were spoken to you with a firm, decided emphasis: 'Put that out of your hand! You need not take that; your life is not your own; your MEDICINE is not needed to bring you peace and rest. What you need is heart religion, a heart purified, refined, elevated from common things, taking hold upon the {162} divine. Be a man. Call your wife to your side, become better acquainted with the truth, be molded by the Spirit of God, and you will have peace. If you take the right course, if you are unwavering in the truth, if you keep your own soul in the love of

God, you will be in the hands of the Lord the means of saving your wife, and in her turn, if she accepts the truth of heavenly origin, if she is a meek and humble follower of Christ, she will be the means in the hands of God of being a great blessing to you."

1888—*Pamphlet 96, Testimonies on the Case of Elder E. P. Daniels,* 53–56.

"You are not always as particular about your words as you should be; you make rash statements. The above declarations are not true. I learn that, to excuse your practice of using WINE, you have stated, so I have been informed, that Brother and Sister White kept WINE in their house, and to your certain knowledge used it. This, like the statement in regard to drinking TEA, is not true. Will you please tell me why you make such rash statements? You claim to be my friend; do you imagine these statements will help my influence among the people? I do not use TEA, either green or black. Not a spoonful has passed my lips for many years, except when crossing the ocean, and once since on this side I took it as a MEDICINE when I was sick and vomiting. In such circumstances it may prove a present relief."
(LP—*Selected Messages,* book 2, 302)

"I did not use TEA when you were with us. I have always {54} used RED CLOVER TOP, as I stated to you. I offered you this and told you it was a good, simple, and wholesome drink. I remember that Sister Ings made TEA for you several times by special request. You said you had a headache and must have something to help it, and you said TEA always had helped you. I told her I did not like to have her do this, for it was contrary to my principles. I asked her where she got the TEA, and she said that a family who were on a camping trip had stopped here and a Mr. Wallace who was not a believer was with them, and the party had TEA and made it for him, and when they had gone the TEA was found here, and she supposed they must have left it. I have not bought a penny's worth of TEA for years. Knowing its influence, I would not dare to use it, except in cases of severe vomiting, when I take it as a MEDICINE, but not as a beverage."
(*Selected Messages,* book 2, 302;
LP—*Counsels on Diet and Foods,* 490)

"I have felt alarmed for you for some time because of your use of TEA and WINES. Of all others, you should touch not, taste not, handle not, anything like TEA, COFFEE, WINE, BEER, BRANDY, or ANY STIMULUS. You are of a nature that you cannot safely use anything of that

order. Your preaching to others is not in harmony with your practice. This is against you, and leaves a doubtful impression upon minds in regard to the ministry. Your case is presented before them, and the supposition in their minds is that other ministers indulge in these things, as you do yourself. To cover and excuse yourself, you have misled others by misstating me. I do not preach one thing and practice another. I do not present to my hearers rules of life for them to follow, while I make an exception in my own case. You are a man {55} who should never use TEA, COFFEE, BRANDY, or WINE. Your nervous temperament will become unduly excited, and be followed by corresponding depression. It is perilous for you to educate your tastes and stimulate your nerves, for you are in serious danger of depending on these STIMULANTS and working upon them. The habit of taking STIMULANTS may become second nature and pave the way for you to become a DRUNKARD. You may start back, and feel bitter towards me because I say these things to you, but let me tell you, you have accustomed yourself to these indulgences because you felt that you must have them for their immediate STIMULATING PROPERTIES.
(MP—*Selected Messages,* book 2, 302)

"I have not tested the WINE that you claim is not intoxicating. I have perhaps used half a pint in all, taking a spoonful with a raw egg, much as I hate the taste of WINE. I would not care, even if I had not solemnly pledged myself not to use WINE as a beverage, to make a daily practice of taking even one teaspoonful with a raw egg, for Satan is at work to encourage the use of TEA, COFFEE, WINE, and BEER, that he may make us dependent upon these things, and encourage our resorting to them frequently, so that our appetite and taste will crave these STIMULANTS. I tell you frankly that you would be much better in nerve and muscle if you made a decided change in your practice, not only in drinking STIMULATING DRINKS, but in eating so largely of meat. The animal powers are strengthened by indulgence in these things, and the moral and spiritual powers are overborne. I am not guilty of drinking ANY TEA except RED CLOVER TOP TEA, and if I loved WINE, TEA, and COFFEE, I would not use these HEALTH-DESTROYING {56} NARCOTICS, for I prize health, and I prize a healthful example in all these things. I want to be a pattern of temperance and of good works to others. Will my brother practice as well as preach temperance in all things? If you do this, I do not believe you will be so changeable in your character. Your words will be more select and well chosen. You will not be careless in regard to your

conversation. You will not be so depressed at one time and so hilarious at another, acting like a boy in place of an ambassador of Jesus Christ. I am seriously troubled for your soul. I know people are unwise in praising you and extolling you; should they read you as God sees you, they could not do this. I know that when you have apparent success you are elated, and you crave praise; and you get it from many, who, if their hearts were right with God, would not speak one word to flatter you. They would understand that it is not safe to pet and praise you, or any other poor, sinful mortal. The Lord is to be exalted by all His creatures. Finite man is not to attract admiration or praise, but do his work in humility."
(MP—*Selected Messages,* book 2, 302; *Counsels on Diet and Foods,* 490)

1889—*Manuscript Releases,* vol. 13, 177–178.

"In their practice, the physicians should seek more and more to lessen the use of DRUGS instead of increasing it. When Dr. A came to the Health Retreat, she laid aside her knowledge and practice of hygiene, and administered the little homeopathic doses for almost every ailment. This was against the light God had given. Thus our people, who had been taught to avoid DRUGS in almost every form, were receiving a different education. I was obliged to tell her that this practice of depending upon MEDICINE, whether in large or small doses, was not in accordance with the principles of health reform. (See Appendix A) The Lord had in His providence given light in regard to the establishment of sanitariums where the sick should be treated upon hygienic principles. The people must be taught to depend on the Lord's remedies, pure air, pure water, and simple, healthful foods.
(FP—*Selected Messages,* book 2, 282)

"Every effort made for the physical and moral health of the people should be based on moral principles. The advocates of reform who are laboring with the glory of God in view will plant their feet firmly upon the principles of hygiene; they will adopt a correct practice. The people need true knowledge. By their wrong habits of life, men and women of this {178} generation are bringing upon themselves untold suffering. Physicians have a work to do to bring about reform by educating the people, that they may understand the laws which govern their physical life. They should know how to eat properly, to work intelligently, to dress healthfully, and should be taught to bring all their habits into harmony with the laws of life and health, and to discard DRUGS. There is a great work to be done. If the principles of health reform are carried out, the work will indeed be as closely allied to that of the third angel's message

Spirit of Prophecy References

as the hand is to the body. . . .

"If they move in God's way, physicians of the same faith will be linked together in a strong brotherhood, aiding one another to reach the highest standard, and devising means to enlighten the people, not encouraging the use of DRUGS, but leading away from DRUG MEDI-CATION. Teach the people how to prevent disease. Tell them to cease rebelling against nature's laws, and by removing every obstruction give her a chance to put forth her very best efforts to set things right. Nature must have a fair chance to employ her healing agencies. We must make earnest efforts to reach a higher platform in regard to the methods of treating the sick. If the light which God has given prevails, if truth overcomes error, advanced steps will be taken in health reform. This must be."

1890—*Christian Temperance and Bible Hygiene*, 13.

"The view held by some that spirituality is a detriment to health, is the sophistry of Satan. The religion of the Bible is not detrimental to the health of either body or mind. The influence of the Spirit of God is the VERY BEST MEDICINE for disease. Heaven is all health; and the more deeply heavenly influences are realized, the more sure will be the recovery of the believing invalid. The true principles of Christianity open before all a source of inestimable happiness. Religion is a continual wellspring, from which the Christian can drink at will, and never exhaust the fountain."
(*Counsels on Health*, 28; *Mind, Character, and Personality*, vol. 2, 411; LP—*The Signs of the Times*, January 27, 1909)

1890—*Christian Temperance and Bible Hygiene*, 17–18.

"The use of TOBACCO is an inconvenient, expensive, uncleanly habit. The teachings of Christ, pointing to purity, self-denial, and temperance, all rebuke this defiling {18} practice. When we think of the long fast that Jesus endured in the wilderness of temptation in order to break the power of appetite over man, we marvel that those who profess to be His followers can indulge in this habit. Is it for the glory of God for men to enfeeble the physical powers, confuse the brain, and yield the will to this NARCOTIC POISON? What right have they to mar the image of God? What says the apostle?—'I beseech you therefore, brethren, by the mercies of God, that ye present your bodies a living sacrifice, holy, acceptable unto God, which is your reasonable service.' Romans 12:1."
(*Temperance*, 62)

Spirit of Prophecy References

1890—*Christian Temperance and Bible Hygiene*, 32, 34–37, 40.

"Many who would hesitate to place LIQUOR to a neighbor's lips, will engage in the raising of HOPS, and thus lend their influence against the temperance cause. I cannot see how, in the light of the law of God, Christians can conscientiously engage in the raising of HOPS or in the manufacture of WINE and CIDER for the market. . . . {34}
(Temperance, 98)

"All these nerve irritants are wearing away the life forces, and the restlessness caused by shattered nerves, the impatience, the mental feebleness, become a warring element, antagonizing to spiritual progress. Then should not those who advocate temperance and reform be awake to counteract the evils of these INJURIOUS DRINKS? In some cases it is as difficult to break up the TEA-and-COFFEE HABIT {35} as it is for the inebriate to discontinue the use of LIQUOR. The money expended for TEA and COFFEE is worse than wasted. They do the user only harm, and that continually. Those who use TEA, COFFEE, OPIUM, and ALCOHOL, may sometimes live to old age, but this fact is no argument in favor of the use of these STIMULANTS. What these persons might have accomplished, but failed to do because of their intemperate habits, the great day of God alone will reveal. . . . {36}
(Temperance, 74; Testimony Studies on Diet and Foods, 145; Counsels on Diet and Foods, 421–422)

"We are already suffering because of the wrong habits of our fathers, and yet how many take a course in every way worse than theirs! OPIUM, TEA, COFFEE, TOBACCO, and LIQUOR are rapidly extinguishing the spark of vitality still left in the race. Every year millions of gallons of INTOXICATING LIQUORS are drank, and millions of dollars are spent for TOBACCO. And the slaves of appetite, while constantly spending their earnings in sensual indulgence, rob their children of food and clothing and the advantages of education. There can never be a right state of society while these evils exist.
(Counsels on Diet and Foods, 423; Testimony Studies on Diet and Foods, 146)

"When the appetite for SPIRITUOUS LIQUOR is indulged, the man voluntarily places to his lips the draught which debases below the level of the brute, him who was made in the image of God. Reason is paralyzed, the intellect is benumbed, the animal passions are excited, and then follow crimes of the most debasing character. How can the user of RUM or TOBACCO give to God an undivided heart? It is impossible. Neither can he love his neighbor as himself. The darling indulgence engrosses all his affections. To gratify his craving for STRONG DRINK, he sells reason {37}

and self-control. He places to his lips that which stupefies the brain, paralyzes the intellect, and makes him a shame and curse to his family, and a terror to all around him. If men would become temperate in all things, if they would touch not, taste not, handle not, TEA, COFFEE, TO-BACCO, WINES, OPIUM, and ALCOHOLIC DRINKS, reason would take the reins of government in her own hands, and hold the appetites and passions under control. . . . {40}
(LP—*Temperance*, 94)

"It is not an easy matter to overcome the appetite for NARCOTICS and STIMULANTS. But in the name of Christ this great victory can be gained. His love for the fallen race was so great that He made an infinite sacrifice to reach them in their degradation, and through His divine power finally elevate them to His throne. But it rests with man whether Christ shall accomplish for him that which He is fully able to do. God cannot work against man's will to save him from Satan's artifices. Man must put forth his human power to resist and conquer at any cost; he must be a coworker with Christ. Then, through the victory that it is his privilege to gain by the all-powerful name of Jesus, he may become an heir of God, and a partaker with Christ of His glory. No drunkard can inherit the kingdom of God; but 'to him that overcometh will I grant to sit with me in my throne, even as I also overcame, and am set down with my Father in his throne.' Revelation 3:21."

1890—*Christian Temperance and Bible Hygiene*, 53–54.

"The apostle Peter understood the relation between the mind and the body, and raised his voice in warning to his brethren: 'Dearly beloved, I beseech you as strangers and pilgrims, abstain from fleshly lusts, which war against {54} the soul.' 1 Peter 2:11. Many regard this text as a warning against licentiousness only; but it has a broader meaning. It forbids every injurious gratification of appetite or passion. Every perverted appetite becomes a warring lust. Appetite was given us for a good purpose, not to become the minister of death by being perverted, and thus degenerating into 'lusts which war against the soul.' Peter's admonition is a most direct and forcible warning against the use of all STIMULANTS and NARCOTICS. These indulgences may well be classed among the lusts that exert a pernicious influence upon moral character."
(*Maranatha*, 81)

1890—*Christian Temperance and Bible Hygiene*, 80.

"Since a healthy state of mind depends upon the normal condition of the vital forces, what care should be exercised that neither STIMULANTS nor NARCOTICS be used! Yet we see that a large number of those who profess to be Christians are using TOBACCO. They deplore the evils of intemperance; yet while speaking against the use of LIQUORS, these very men will eject the juice of TOBACCO. There must be a change of sentiment with reference to TOBACCO USING before the root of the evil will be reached. We press the subject still closer. TEA and COFFEE are fostering the appetite for STRONGER STIMULANTS. And then we come still closer home, to the preparation of food, and ask, Is temperance practiced in all things? are the reforms which are essential to health and happiness carried out here?"

(*Counsels on Diet and Foods*, 426–427; *Fundamentals of Christian Education*, 144; *Christian Education*, 181; *Testimony Studies on Diet and Foods*, 146, 156)

1890—*Christian Temperance and Bible Hygiene*, 100–101.

"When the weather will permit, those who are engaged in sedentary occupations, should, if possible, walk out in {101} the open air every day, summer and winter. The clothing should be suitable, and the feet well protected. Walking is often more beneficial to health than all the MEDICINE that can be prescribed. For those who can endure it, walking is preferable to riding; for it brings all the muscles into exercise. The lungs also are forced into healthy action, since it is impossible to walk in the bracing air of a winter morning without inflating them."

1890—*Christian Temperance and Bible Hygiene*, 121.

"A great amount of good can be done by enlightening all to whom we have access, as to the best means, not only of curing the sick, but of preventing disease and suffering. The physician who endeavors to enlighten his patients as to the nature and causes of their maladies, and to teach them how to avoid disease, may have uphill work; but if he is a conscientious reformer, he will talk plainly of the ruinous effects of self-indulgence in eating, drinking, and dressing, of the overtaxation of the vital forces that has brought his patients where they are. He will not increase the evil by administering DRUGS till exhausted nature gives up the struggle, but will teach the patients how to form correct habits, and to aid nature in her work of restoration by a wise use of her own simple remedies."

(*Healthful Living*, 248; *Testimony Studies on Diet and Foods*, 114; *Counsels on Health*, 451–452; *Counsels on Diet and Foods*, 449)

Spirit of Prophecy References

1890—*Christian Temperance and Bible Hygiene*, 132–133.

"But few of the youth are free from corruption. Impure habits are practiced to an alarming extent, and have done more than any other evil to cause the degeneration of the race. Children who indulge secret vice are {133} often puny and dwarfed. The anxious parents seek a physician, and DRUGS are administered; but the evil is not removed, for the cause still exists."

1890—*Medical Ministry*, 230–231.

"If we neglect to do that which is within the reach of nearly every family, and ask the Lord to relieve pain when we are too indolent to make use of these remedies within our power, it is simply presumption. The Lord expects us to work in order that we may obtain food. He does not propose that we shall gather the harvest unless we break the sod, till the soil, and cultivate the produce. Then God sends the rain and the sunshine and the clouds to cause vegetation to flourish. God works and man cooperates with God. Then there is seedtime and harvest. God has caused to grow out of the ground HERBS for the use of man, and if we understand the nature of these ROOTS and HERBS, and {231} make a right use of them, there would not be a necessity of running for the doctor so frequently, and people would be in much better health than they are today."

(LP—*Pamphlet 144, The Place of Herbs in Rational Therapy, 7*)

1890—*Medical Ministry*, 259–260.

"God's blessing will rest upon every effort made to awaken an interest in health reform; for it is needed everywhere. There must be a revival on this subject; for God purposes to accomplish much through this agency. Present temperance with all its advantages in reference to health. Educate people in the laws of life so that they may know how to preserve health. The efforts actually put forth at present are not meeting the mind of God. DRUG MEDICATION is a curse to this enlightened age.

"Educate away from DRUGS. Use them less and less, and depend more upon hygienic agencies; then nature will respond to God's physicians—pure air, pure water, proper exercise, a clear conscience.

"Many might recover without one grain of MEDICINE, if they would live out the laws of health. DRUGS need seldom be used. {260} It will require earnest, patient, protracted effort to establish the work and to carry it forward upon hygienic principles. But let fervent prayer and faith be combined with your efforts, and you will succeed. By this work you will be teaching the patients, and others also, how to take care of themselves when sick, without resorting to the use of DRUGS."

1890—*Medical Ministry, 263–264.*

"The minds of the suffering ones must be led to grasp the hope of deliverance from special peril. Speak to them hopeful words, words of courage. There are those patronizing our sanitariums {264} whom the Lord will heal if they will abstain from the use of LIQUOR and DRUGS and will use simple and safe remedies to counteract disease brought on through perverted appetite. If they will act their part to break the spell of the enemy by firmly resisting temptation, and will surrender themselves to the One who gave His life for sinful souls, they will become sons and daughters of God."

1890—*Pamphlet 66, Health, Philanthropic, and Medical Missionary Work, 43.*

"Among the greatest dangers to our health institutions is the influence of physicians, superintendents, and helpers who profess to believe the present truth, but who have never taken their stand fully upon health reform. Some have no conscientious scruples in regard to their eating, drinking, and dressing. How can the physician or anyone else present the matter as it is when he himself is indulging in the use of harmful things? God's blessing will rest upon every effort made to awaken an interest in health reform; for it is needed everywhere. There must be a revival in regard to this matter; for God purposes to accomplish much through this agency. DRUG MEDICATION, as it is generally practiced, is a curse. Educate away from DRUGS. Use them less and less, and depend more upon hygienic agencies; then nature will respond to God's physicians—pure air, pure water, proper exercise, a clear conscience. Those who persist in the use of TEA, COFFEE, and flesh meats will feel the need of DRUGS, but many might recover without one grain of MEDICINE if they would obey the laws of health. DRUGS need seldom be used." (*Counsels on Health*, 26;.

LP—*Selected Messages*, book 2, 281–283; *Medical Ministry*, 259; *Temperance*, 85; *Healthful Living*, 246–247; *General Conference Daily Bulletin*, January 30, 1893)

1890—*The Paulson Collection of Ellen G. White Letters, 28–29.*

"Now in regard to that which we can do for ourselves. There is a point that requires careful, thoughtful consideration. I must become acquainted with myself, I must be a learner always as to how to take care of this building, the body God has given me, that I may preserve it in the very best condition of health. I must eat those things which will be for my very best good physically, and I must take special care to have my clothing such as will conduce to a healthful circulation of the blood. I must not deprive myself of exercise and air. I must get all the sunlight that it is possible for me to obtain. I must have wisdom to be a faithful guardian of my body. I should do a very unwise thing to enter a cool room when in a perspiration; I should show myself an unwise steward to allow myself to sit in a draught, {29} and thus expose myself so as to take cold. I should be unwise to sit with cold feet and limbs and thus drive back the blood from the extremities to the brain or internal organs. I should always protect my feet in damp weather. I should eat regularly of the most healthful food which will make the best quality of blood, and I should not work intemperately if it is in my power to avoid doing so. And when I violate the laws God has established in my being, I am to repent and reform, and place myself in the most favorable condition under the doctors God has provided—pure air, pure water, and the healing, precious sunlight. Water can be used in many ways to relieve suffering. Draughts of clear, hot water, taken before eating (half a quart, more or less), will never do any harm, but will rather be productive of good. A cup of TEA made from CATNIP HERB will quiet the nerves. HOP TEA will induce sleep. HOP POULTICES over the stomach will relieve pain. If the eyes are weak, if there is pain in the eyes, or inflammation, soft flannel clothes wet in hot water and salt, will bring relief quickly. When the head is congested, if the feet and limbs are put in a bath with a little MUSTARD, relief will be obtained. There are many more simple remedies which will do much to restore healthful action to the body. All these simple preparations the Lord expects us to use for ourselves, but man's extremities are God's opportunities. If we neglect to do that which is within the reach of nearly every family, and ask the Lord to relieve pain, when we are too indolent to make use of these remedies within our power, it is simply presumption. The Lord expects us to work in order that we obtain food. He does not propose that we shall gather the harvest unless we break the sod, till the soil, and cultivate the produce. Then God sends the rain and the sunshine and the clouds to cause vegetation to flourish. God works and man cooperates with God. Then there is seedtime

Spirit of Prophecy References

and harvest. God has caused to grow out of the ground, HERBS for the use of man, and if we understand the nature of those ROOTS and HERBS, and make a right use of them, there would not be a necessity of running for the doctor, so frequently, and people would be in much better health than they are today. I believe in calling upon the Great Physician when we have used the remedies I have mentioned. In regard to manner of labor, we certainly need to be wise as serpents and harmless as doves. We might be very zealous, but it might be an unwise zeal, and serve to hedge up our way. Then there is danger of being so circumscribed in our work as to do very little good."
(*Pamphlet 144, The Place of Herbs in Rational Therapy,* 5–7; FP—*Selected Messages,* book 2, 296–298)

1891—*Pamphlet 66, Health, Philanthropic, and Medical Missionary Work,* 36–37.

"Neglect of prayer causes the Christian to become weak, to lose self-control, to give rein to impure thoughts and impulses. But in learning of Christ, in looking to Jesus, in depending upon his strength, the physician will be brought into sympathy with Christ; and in treating the sick he will seek God for wisdom. Then instead of placing his dependence upon DRUGS, and expecting that MEDICINE will bring health to his patients, he will use nature's restoratives, and employ natural means whereby the sick may be aided to recovery. The Lord will hear and answer the prayer of the Christian physician, and he may reach an elevated standard if he will but lay hold upon the hand of Christ, and determine that he will not let go. Golden opportunities are open to the Christian physician; for he may exert a precious influence upon those with whom he is brought in contact. He may guide and mold and fashion the lives of his patients by holding before them heavenly principles. The physician should let men see that he does not regard his work as of a cheap order, but looks upon it as high, noble, elevated work, even that to which is attached the sacred accountability of dealing with both the {37} souls and the bodies of those for whom Christ has paid the infinite price of his most precious blood. If the physician has the mind of Christ, he will be cheerful, hopeful, and happy, but not trifling. He will realize that heavenly angels accompany him to the sickroom, and will find words to speak readily, truthfully, to his patients, that will cheer and bless them. His faith will be full of simplicity, of childlike confidence in the Lord. He will be able to repeat to the repenting soul the gracious promises of God, and thus place the trembling hand of the afflicted ones in the hand of Christ, that they may find repose in God. Thus, through the grace imparted to him, the physician will fulfill his Heavenly Father's claims upon him. In delicate and perilous operations he may know that Jesus is by his side to counsel, to strengthen, to nerve him to act with precision and skill in his efforts to save human life. If the presence of God is not in the sickroom, Satan will be there to suggest perilous experiments, and will seek to unbalance the nerves, so that life will be destroyed rather than saved."

1891—*Temperance*, 273–274.

"Would that the Fall of Adam and Eve had been the only fall; but from the loss of Eden to the present time, there has been a succession of falls. Satan has planned to ruin man, by leading him away from loyalty to the commandments of God, and one of his most successful methods is that of tempting him to the gratification of perverted appetite. We see on all sides the marks of man's intemperance. In our cities and villages the {274} saloon is on every corner, and in the countenances of its patrons we see the dreadful work of ruin and destruction. On every side, Satan seeks to entice the youth into the path of perdition; and if he can once get their feet set in the way, he hurries them on in their downward course, leading them from one dissipation to another, until his victims lose their tenderness of conscience, and have no more the fear of God before their eyes. They exercise less and less self-restraint. They become addicted to the use of WINE and ALCOHOL, TOBACCO, and OPIUM, and go from one stage of debasement to another. They are slaves to appetite. Counsel which they once respected, they learn to despise. They put on swaggering airs, and boast of liberty when they are the servants of corruption. They mean by liberty that they are slaves to selfishness, debased appetite, and licentiousness."
(*Mind, Character, and Personality,* vol.1, 76; *Maranatha,* 139)

1891—*Temperance*, 278.

"Those also who use TOBACCO are weakening their physical and mental power. The use of TOBACCO has no foundation in nature. Nature rebels against the NARCOTIC, and when the TOBACCO USER first tries to force this unnatural habit upon the system, a hard battle is fought. The stomach, and, indeed, the whole system, revolts against the abominable practice, but the evildoer perseveres until nature gives up the struggle, and the man becomes a SLAVE OF TOBACCO."

Spirit of Prophecy References

1892—*Healthful Living,* 247.

"To use DRUGS while continuing evil habits is certainly inconsistent, and greatly dishonors God by dishonoring the body which he has made. Yet for all this, STIMULANTS and DRUGS continue to be prescribed and freely used; while the hurtful indulgences that produce the disease are not discarded. The use of TEA, COFFEE, TOBACCO, OPIUM, WINE, BEER, and other STIMULANTS gives nature a false support. Physicians should understand how to treat the sick through the use of nature's remedies. Pure air, pure water, and healthful exercise should be employed in the treatment of the sick."

1892—*Manuscript Releases,* vol. 16, 57–59.

"All that you have written in your last letter I read with great interest. That which you say in regard to the matter of physicians having professional badges, I fully endorse. Christian physicians need no badge except that of Christianity. The use of DRUGS is not in accordance with God's plan. Physicians should understand how to treat the sick through the use of nature's remedies. Pure air, pure water, healthful exercise, should be employed in the treatment of the sick. . . . {58}

"Many indulge in unhealthful practices until the physical vitality is undermined, and the mental and moral powers are enfeebled. When they fall a prey to disease they resort to DRUGS, and if these afford them temporary {59} relief, they seem to be satisfied to continue in transgression. They do not bring their habits and practices in review to see what is wrong, and correct the evils by removing the causes. As the DRUGS are a mere STIMULANT, after a time they realize that they are in a worse condition than before they used the remedies. To use DRUGS while continuing evil habits, is certainly inconsistent, and greatly dishonors God by dishonoring the body which He has made. Yet for all this, STIMULANTS and DRUGS continue to be prescribed and freely used by human beings, while the hurtful indulgences that produced the disease are not discarded. They use TEA, COFFEE, TOBACCO, OPIUM, WINE, BEER, and other STIMULANTS and give to nature a false support."
(MP—*Temperance,* 84)

1892—*Manuscript Releases,* vol. 19, 227.

"When Edson and Willie were very sick, we first prayed earnestly to God that He would rebuke the disease and heal them. Then did we feel relieved from doing everything in our power for their recovery? No. We worked most vigorously, using God's own remedies. We applied water in various ways, praying the Lord to accept our efforts and give us strength and wisdom to use (not DRUG MEDICATION) but the simple, natural remedies God had provided. Thus we were cooperating with God."

1892—*Manuscript Releases,* vol. 19, 297.

"Last night I spent many wakeful hours in prayer. I am resolved to cast myself, body, soul, and spirit, upon the Lord. I cannot take DRUGS. They do me no good, but harm. I long for the blessing of the Lord. My heart goes out after God. I tremble at His word. I am encouraged as I look to Jesus and recount His loving kindnesses: 'In my distress I called upon the Lord, and cried unto my God: he heard my voice out of his temple, and my cry came before him, even into his ears.' 'He brought me forth also into a large place; he delivered me, because he delighted in me.' Psalm 18:6, 19. 'I love the Lord, because he hath heard my voice and my supplications.' Psalms 116:1. This has been my experience day and night during my sickness."

1892—*The Use of Drugs in the Care of the Sick,* Ellen G. White Publications Manuscript, 42–43.

"In regard to hygienic methods and the disuse of DRUGS, from the light God has given me, there must be a reform. Our people are going far from the light which God has given on this subject. If Dr. B or Dr. A or any other doctor goes into the institutions, he must work in harmony with the light God has seen fit to give to His people in reform methods of treatment. If Dr. A and his wife unite with Dr. B. or any other physician, all egotism must be done away. The spirit that controlled the medical fraternity has been of that character which will exclude many from heaven unless they put away this spirit and work with the mind and spirit of Christ. Wicked jealousies, evil thinking, evil speaking of their brethren, has been an offense to God. The methods of DRUG MEDICATION have created the bitterest animosity in feeling, almost equal to the prejudice that Catholics have manifested toward Protestants because they did not view every point of religious faith as they themselves.

"Such a spirit may be expected in the world, but when it becomes a controlling power among Christians, it is an offense to God. It is a shame when a reform among the medical fraternity or the church will be purged from those who will not be Bible Christians. It is altogether too late in the day for such a Satanic exhibition of spirit as is revealed among medical DRUG PRACTITIONERS. God abhors it. I could write much on this subject, but I am not able now.

1892—*Manuscript Releases*, vol. 20, 122.

"Lead them away from DRUG MEDICATION, educating them and training them that DRUGS kill more than they cure. This matter is presented to me so frequently that I cannot hold my peace upon this subject. The use of POISONOUS DRUGS is coming more and more into practice among our people. The light which the Lord has given me is that institutions should be established to do away with DRUGS, and use God's agencies; that instruction should be given daily upon this subject. But God's ways and instruction have not been heeded, therefore not one-twentieth part of the good has been accomplished which might have been if Christian physicians had heeded the admonitions and the counsel of the Most High."

1892—*Manuscript Releases*, vol. 20, 394.

"The use of DRUGS in our institutions, to the extent to which they are used, is a libel upon the name of hygienic institutions for the treatment of the sick. The physicians need to be converted on this point as decidedly as the sinner needs the converting power of God on life and character in order to become a pure-hearted Christian. Let the students who go to obtain a medical education at the medical institutes of our land learn all that they possibly can of the principles of life, but let them discard error, and not become bigots. I would not speak thus plainly unless I felt that it was necessary."

1892—*Spalding and Magan Collection*, 7.

"The use of DRUGS has not been specified as in the Lord's order, but He has given special light concerning our health institutions, directing His people to practice and cultivate hygienic principles. Such should be taught those who are in ignorance as to how to live in accordance with pure principles, practicing those things that will preserve the body in a healthy condition. Man is to cooperate with God-given ability. He is not to be ignorant as to what are right practices in eating and drinking, and in all his habits of life. The Lord designs that His human agents shall act as rational, accountable beings in every respect."

Spirit of Prophecy References

1893—*The Ellen G. White Biography*, 1891–1900, vol. 4, 106.

"I spoke upon temperance, and this is a living question here at this time. Hundreds were out to hear, and there was perfect order. . . . Mothers and any number of children were present. You would have supposed that the children had had an OPIATE, for there was not a whimper from them. My voice reached all over the enclosure (paddock is the name they give it here)."

1893—*Manuscript Releases*, vol. 8, 85–86.

"After the teeth were extracted Sister Caro shook like an aspen leaf. Her hands were shaking and she was suffering pain of body. She had felt sick, she said, on the cars during her ten hours' ride. She dreaded to give pain to Sister White. She slept little Tuesday night and could scarcely eat in the morning, but she knew she must perform the operation and went through with it. Then the patient waited upon the doctor; I had her seated in my easy chair and gave her sips of CHOLERA MIXTURE [a NOSTRUM used for intestinal disorders]—all the STUMULUS I had in the house. . . . {86}

"I thank my heavenly Father I bore the trial without a groan and in the use of my senses. I took nothing to stupefy me, and as the result have not the influence of STUPEFYING DRUGS to recover from. I am pleased to bid farewell to these teeth that have caused me so great suffering. I have expended no less than one hundred and fifty dollars on them and endured very much pain."

1893—*Selected Messages*, book 2, 278–280.

Seventh-day Adventist Medical Student—"From our study of the *Testimonies* and the little work, *How to Live*, we can see that the Lord is strongly opposed to the use of drugs in our medical work. . . . Several of the students are in doubt as to the meaning of the word 'DRUG' as mentioned in *How to Live*. Does it refer only to the STRONGER MEDICINES as MERCURY, STRYCHNINE, ARSENIC, and such POISONS, the things we medical students call 'DRUGS,' or does it also include the simpler remedies, as POTASSIUM, IODINE, SQUILLS, and so on? We know that our success will be proportionate to our adherence to God's methods. For this reason I have asked the above question."

Ellen G. White—"Your questions, I will say, are answered largely, if not definitely, in *How to Live*. DRUG POISONS mean the articles which you have mentioned. The simpler remedies are less harmful in proportion to their simplicity; but in very many cases these are used when not at all necessary. There are SIMPLE HERBS and ROOTS that every family may use for themselves and need not call a physician any sooner than they would call a lawyer. I do not think that I can give you any definite line of MEDI-CINES compounded and dealt out by doctors, that are perfectly harmless. And yet it would not be wisdom to engage in controversy over this subject. *(Pamphlet 144, The Place of Herbs in Rational Therapy, 8)*

"The practitioners are very much in earnest in using their DAN-GEROUS CONCOCTIONS, and I am decidedly opposed to resorting to such things. They never cure; they may change the difficulty to create a worse one. Many of those who practice the prescribing of DRUGS, would not take the same or give them to their children. If they have an intelligent knowledge of the human body, if they understand the delicate, wonderful human machinery, they must know {280} that we are fearfully and wonderfully made, and that not a particle of these STRONG DRUGS should be introduced into this human living organism. *(Pamphlet 144, The Place of Herbs in Rational Therapy, 8)*

"As the matter was laid open before me, and the sad burden of the result of DRUG MEDICATION, the light was given me that Seventh-day Adventists should establish health institutions discarding all these HEALTH-DESTROYING INVENTIONS, and physicians should treat the sick upon hygienic principles. The great burden should be to have well-trained nurses, and well-trained medical practitioners to educate 'precept upon precept; line upon line, line upon line; here a little, and there a little.' Isaiah. 28:10." *(Pamphlet 144, The Place of Herbs in Rational Therapy, 8–9)*

1893—*Sermons and Talks*, vol. 1, 217.

"God has given us reasoning powers and talents of perception that we may distinguish between good and evil. This we may do if we refuse to yield to the temptations of Satan, who is playing the game of life for every soul. But if we stupefy our faculties by the use of NAR-COTICS, we cannot distinguish between right and wrong, between the sacred and the common. The sin of this lies at our own door. We have given our powers into Satan's keeping, and habits that are selfish and impure bind us as with chains of steel.

1893—*Spalding and Magan Collection*, 85.

"We cannot attach our names to a pledge presented by a society which indulges the use of the body-and-soul-destroying NARCOTIC,

Spirit of Prophecy References

TOBACCO. How can we unite with this class, how work with them, how form a society with them? How is it possible to work successfully in their way and after their order?"

1893—*Temperance*, 60.

"In fastening upon men the terrible habit of TOBACCO USING, it is Satan's purpose to palsy the brain and confuse the judgment, so that sacred things shall not be discerned. When once an appetite for this NARCOTIC has been formed, it takes firm hold of the mind and the will of man, and he is in bondage under its power. Satan has the control of the will, and eternal realities are eclipsed. Man cannot stand forth in his God-given manhood; he is a slave to perverted appetite."

1893—*Temperance*, 105.

"The TOBACCO HABIT . . . beclouds so many minds. Why do you not give up this habit? Why not arise and say, I will serve sin and the devil no longer? Say, I will let alone this POISONOUS NARCOTIC. You never can do it in your own strength. Christ says, 'I am at thy right hand to help thee.' "

1894—*The Ellen G. White Biography*, 1891–1900, vol. 4, 119.

"As a denomination we are in the fullest sense total abstainers from the use of SPIRITUOUS LIQUORS, WINE, BEER, CIDER, and also TOBACCO and all NARCOTICS, and are earnest workers in the cause of temperance. All are vegetarians, many abstaining wholly from the use of flesh food, while others use it in only the most moderate degree."

1894—*Manuscript Releases*, vol. 8, 144–145.

"Willie has been having a long siege of council meetings and committee meetings. While pitching our tents, in driving a stake, he missed his stroke or his finger got in the way of the iron sledge, and he smashed his finger, splitting open the flesh to the bone in three places, but not breaking the {145} bone. The nail had to be drawn out. This finger needed considerable care. Brother Simmons dressed it carefully every day, but as this finger difficulty was in a fair way of recovery, a small pimple appeared on his wrist which increased to great inflammation, and after more than one week of suffering, the core came out and the second gathering appeared. HOPS [POULTICES] and Elder Blow soon brought that to a head, and he now has some peace. He concluded to take my span of horses and platform wagon and Brother McKenzie and himself came to this place."

Spirit of Prophecy References

1894—Sermons and Talks, vol. 2, 106.

"What is your practice? Are you injuring your understanding through using NARCOTICS, TOBACCO, WINE, and LIQUOR? I warn you of that path because God warns you all from it. You must give a good example to your children. It was sin that brought the agony upon the Son of the infinite God, taking the wrath of God upon His own divine soul. What hereditary trusts have you gathered? Have you gathered them up from Abel, Noah, Abraham? God says of Abraham, 'I know him, that he will command his children and his household after him.' Genesis 18:19."

1896—Healthful Living, 248.

"The question of health reform is not agitated as it must be and will be. A simple diet and the entire absence of DRUGS, leaving nature free to recuperate the wasted energies of the body, would make our sanitariums far more effectual in restoring the sick to health."
(*Counsels on Diet and Foods*, 304; *Temperance*, 89; *Testimony Studies on Diet and Foods*, 84; *Spalding and Magan Collection*, 41)

1896—Healthful Living, 264.

"When physicians understand physiology in its truest sense, their use of DRUGS will be very much less, and finally they will cease to use them at all. The physician who depends upon DRUG MEDICATION in his practice shows that he does not understand the delicate machinery of the human organism."

1896—Manuscript Releases, vol. 10, 287.

" 'Died because of bad cooking.' 'Died because of sour bread.' 'Died of MEDICATION.' 'Died of an abused stomach.' This might be written over the graves of many. This suicidal process is gradual. Nature bears the abuse as long as possible, but in the end she must succumb. The oil in the lamp of life is mixed with a variety of INJURIOUS SUBSTANCES, and the lamp refuses to burn longer. It is extinguished, not because God willed it, but because of the manifest disregard of nature's laws."
(*Manuscript Releases*, vol. 14, 299–300)

1896—Medical Ministry, 229.

"When you understand physiology in its truest sense, your DRUG BILLS will be very much smaller, and finally you will cease to deal out DRUGS at all. The physician who depends upon DRUG MEDICATION in his practice shows that he does not understand the delicate machinery of the human organism. He is introducing into the system a seed crop

that will never lose its destroying properties throughout the lifetime. I
tell you this because I dare not withhold it. Christ paid too much for
man's redemption to have his body so ruthlessly treated as it has been
by DRUG MEDICATION.
(*Selected Messages,* book 2, 283–284)

"Years ago the Lord revealed to me that institutions should be established for treating the sick without DRUGS. Man is God's property, and the
ruin that has been made of the living habitation, the suffering caused by the
seeds of death sown in the human system, are an offense to God."
(*Manuscript Releases,* vol. 20, 117–118)

1896—*Selected Messages,* book 2, 113.

"The hardest task I ever had to do in this line was in dealing with
one who, I knew, wanted to follow the Lord. For some time he had
thought he was obtaining new light. He was very ill, and must soon
die. And oh, how my heart hoped he would not make it necessary
for me to tell him just what he was doing. Those to whom he presented his views listened to him eagerly, and some thought him inspired. He had a chart made, and reasoned from the Scriptures to
show that the Lord would come at a certain date, in 1894, I think. To
many his reasoning seemed to be without a flaw. They told of his
powerful exhortations in his sickroom. Most wonderful views passed
before him. But what was the source of his inspiration? It was the
MORPHINE given him to relieve his pain."
(*Manuscript Releases,* vol. 17, 16;
F & LP—*Maranatha,* 233)

1896—*Spalding and Magan Collection,* 30–31.

"There are those associated with you that should ever have kept
before them their aptness and inclination to use POISONOUS DRUGS, that
{31} kill if they do not relieve. The light that God has given upon the
subject of disease and its causes, needs to be dwelt upon largely for it is
the wrong habit of indulgence of appetite and careless, reckless inattention to properly care for the body that tells upon the people. Habits of
cleanliness, [and] care in regard to that which is introduced into the
mouth, should be observed."

1896—*Spalding and Magan Collection,* 44–45.

"My brother, there is need that economy be practiced in every
line of our work. There is need of prayer, earnest, heartfelt, sincere
prayer. There is need that temperance in eating, drinking and build-

ing shall be practiced. There is need to educate the people in right habits of living. Put no confidence in DRUG MEDICINE. If every particle of it were buried in the great ocean, I would say Amen. Our physicians are not working on the right plan. A reform is needed which will go deeper and be more {45} thorough. Meat eating is doing its work, for the meat is diseased. We may not long be able to use even milk. The very earth is groaning under the corrupted inhabitants. We need to consider closely our habits and practices, and banish our sinful, darling indulgences. I have had light from God on this subject, and I have been endeavoring to give this light to our people in this country. I could write you pages upon pages of this; but I feel so deeply over these things that I scarcely dare to take my pen in my hands."

1896—*Temperance*, 88–89.

"Our institutions are established that the sick may be treated by hygienic methods, discarding almost entirely the use of DRUGS. . . . There is a terrible account to be rendered to God by men who have so little regard for human life as to treat the body so ruthlessly in dealing out their DRUGS. . . . We are not excusable if through ignorance we destroy God's building by taking into our stomachs POISONOUS DRUGS under a variety of names we do not understand. It is our duty to refuse all such PRESCRIPTIONS. We wish to build a sanitarium where maladies may be cured by nature's own provisions, and where the people may be taught how to treat themselves when sick; where they will learn to eat temperately of wholesome food, and be educated to refuse all NARCOTICS—TEA, COFFEE, FERMENTED {89} WINES, and STIMULANTS of all kinds—and to discard the flesh of dead animals."

(*Selected Messages*, book 2, 283; *Healthful Living*, 246;
LP—*Counsels on Diet and Foods*, 281; *Testimony Studies on Diet and Foods*, 149)

1897—*The Ellen G. White Biography*, 1891–1900, vol. 4, 293–294.

"Brother Herbert walked from his father's to the meeting in {294} the new building. He feels so well and we are so very thankful that the Lord wrought in his behalf, making Brother Semmens His human agent. He carried through the case without DRUGS. (See Appendix A) W. C. White, the Lord has opened to me why so many cases are lost who have typhoid fever. They are DRUGGED, and nature has not strength to overcome the DRUGS given them."

Spirit of Prophecy References

1897—*The Ellen G. White Biography*, 1891–1900, vol. 4, 309.

"I feel very sad when I consider that young men come from Battle Creek with a deficient education in spiritual godliness. After devoting years of study in the school at Battle Creek, some have stated they had an education that was of little use to them. I see more and more the folly of five years in succession devoted to the education of any student. Let them learn common hard work, in exercising the muscles and their hands, and let them learn from books that have not one grain of infidelity sprinkled in through their brilliant productions. It is like the sugarcoated pills that are used—a DRUG to destroy rather than to restore."

1897—*General Conference Daily Bulletin*, March 2, 1897.

"All nature makes manifest the work of God. Man is fearfully and wonderfully made, and if man had obeyed the laws of Jehovah in his natural laws, the image of God would have been revealed in him. But by sinning against his own body; by indulging his natural appetite and disturbing the action of the human machinery; by the use of ALCOHOLIC DRINKS, NARCOTICS, and the flesh of diseased animals, man has distorted and crippled the Lord's divine arrangements. Nature does her best to expel the POISONOUS DRUG, TOBACCO, but frequently she is overborne. She gives up her struggle to expel the intruder, and the life is sacrificed in the conflict. Every PERNICIOUS DRUG placed in the human stomach, whether by prescription of physician, or by man himself doing violence to the human organism, injures the whole machinery. Every intemperate indulgence or lustful appetite is at war with natural instinct, and the healthful condition of every nerve and muscle and organ of the wonderful human machinery which through the Creator's power possesses organic life.

(*The Paulson Collection of Ellen G. White Letters*, 164–165;
MP—*Selected Messages*, book 2, 280–281; *Temperance*, 57; *Healthful Living*, 109)

"Nature would do her work wisely and well if the human agent would, in his treatment of the body, cooperate with the divine purpose. But how Satan and his whole confederacy rejoice to see how easily his power of deception and art can persuade man to form an appetite for most unpleasant STIMULANTS and NARCOTICS. And then when nature has been overborne, enfeebled in all her working force, there is the DRUG MEDICATION to come from the physician, to kill the remaining vital force, and leave men miserable wrecks of suffering, of imbecility, of insanity, and of loathsome disease. God is hidden from the human

observation by the hellish shadow of Satan."
(*The Paulson Collection of Ellen G. White Letters,* 165)

1897—*Manuscript Releases,* vol. 20, 2.

"You say again, 'They are not educated in regard to the injurious effects of meat eating and of using sugar and vinegar, TEA and COFFEE. That is, they depend for their HERB DRINK on TEA from China and COFFEE from Java. These things are injurious and deleterious to the human system. TEA and COFFEE are STIMULANTS and POISONS, and their effects have been presented before them.' "

1897—*Manuscript Releases,* vol. 20, 36.

"In regard to the book on Christian temperance, that portion that was expressed in reference to DRUG MEDICATION as though it was recommended by me is not according to the light that I have been given to present to the people. I must, if I made this statement, have done so in expressing the idea of working away from the use of all DRUGS concocted at the apothecary. We have no use for them. We should not vindicate the use of DRUG MEDICATION. I did not wish to prejudice the medical fraternity that I could not in my writings approach them, therefore have kept quite silent in reference to the sharp points which I can express. If it is thought that the sentence will not misstate my position, let it stand. But if, knowing of my true position in reference to DRUG MEDICATION, any statements in the book contradict it, would be making me to say Yea, and Nay. I do not know as that expression will do any particular harm, but would rather it would have been left out. This is a reform which will be made by Seventh-day Adventist practitioners. I feel deeply over every matter on which warnings have been given us."

1897—*Manuscript Releases,* vol. 21, 289–291.

"I have read the manuscript Willie sent me for the book *Christian Temperance.* I see nothing that I object to except the subject of DRUG MEDICATION. As matters have been opened to me from time to time, as I have been conducted through the rooms of the sick in the sanitarium and out of the sanitarium, I have seen that the physicians of the sanitarium, by practicing DRUG MEDICATION, have lost many cases that need not have died if they had left their DRUGS out of the sickroom. Cases have been lost that had the physicians left off entirely their DRUG TREATMENT, had they put their wits to work and wisely and persistently used the Lord's own remedies—plenty of air and water—the fever cases that have been lost would have recovered. The reckless use of those things that should be discarded has decided the case of the sick.

"I will not educate or sustain the use of DRUGS. I try not to speak of these things, but if the book is already out, I shall have to insert something that I may place the truth of the matter before the people. After seeing so much harm done by the administering of DRUGS, I cannot use them, and cannot testify in their favor. I must be true to the light given me by the Lord. (LP—*Selected Messages,* book 2, 293)

"The treatment we gave when the sanitarium was first established required earnest labor to combat disease. We did not use DRUG CON- COCTIONS; we followed hygienic methods. This work was blessed by God. It was a work in which the human instrumentality could cooperate with God in saving life. There should be nothing put into the human system that would leave its baleful influence behind. And to carry out the light on this subject, to practice hygienic treatment, and to educate on altogether different lines of treating the sick, was the reason given me why we should have sanitariums established in various localities. (*Selected Messages,* book 2, 293)

"I have been pained when many students have been encouraged to go to Ann Arbor to receive an education in the use of DRUGS. The light which I have received has placed an altogether different complexion on {290} the use made of DRUGS than is given at Ann Arbor or at the sanitarium. We must become enlightened on these subjects. The intri- cate names given the MEDICINES are used to cover up the matter, so that none will know what is given them as remedies unless they obtain a dictionary to find out the meaning of these names. (*Selected Messages,* book 2, 293–294)
LP—*Pamphlet 144, The Place of Herbs in Rational Therapy,* 9)

"The Lord has given some SIMPLE HERBS of the field that at times are beneficial; and if every family were educated in how to use these HERBS in case of sickness, much suffering might be prevented, and no doctor need be called. These old fashioned SIMPLE HERBS, used intelli- gently, would have recovered many sick who have died under DRUG MEDICATION.
(*Selected Messages,* book 2, 294; *Pamphlet 144, The Place of Herbs in Rational Therapy,* 9)

"One of the most beneficial remedies is PULVERIZED CHARCOAL, placed in a bag and used in fomentations. This is a most successful remedy. If wet in SMARTWEED boiled, it is still better. I have ordered this in cases where the sick were suffering great pain, and when it has been confided to me by the physician that he thought it was the last before the close of life. Then I suggested the CHARCOAL, and the patient slept, the turning point came, and recovery was the result. (*Pamphlet 144, The Place of Herbs in Rational Therapy, 24; Selected Messages,* book 2, 294)

"To students when injured with bruised hands and suffering with inflammation, I have prescribed this simple remedy, with perfect success. The POISON of inflammation was overcome, the pain removed, and healing went on rapidly. The most severe inflammation of the eyes will be relieved by a POULTICE of CHARCOAL, put in a bag, and dipped in hot or cold water, as will best suit the case. This works like a charm. (*Pamphlet 144, The Place of Herbs in Rational Therapy, 24*)

"I expect you will laugh at this, but if I could give this remedy some outlandish name that no one knew but myself, it would have greater influence. But Dr. Kellogg, many things have been opened before me that no one but myself is any the wiser for in regard to the management of sickness and disease—the effect of the use of DRUG MEDICATION, the thousands in our work who might have lived if they had not sent for a physician and had let nature work the recovery herself. But the simplest remedies may assist nature, and leave no baleful effects after their use.

I have been studying my own case. I have not applied to any physician since living in this country. I did pay four pounds the first year for electric baths, which did me no good. If indisposed I would just as soon think of calling in a lawyer as a physician.

I have recently left off the use of all liquids, such as homemade COFFEE, with my meals. I eat my food as dry as possible. The result is excellent. In the morning I take lemon and water. I drink nothing between meals unless it be occasionally some lemon and water. At the table I do not eat many things either. I use dry peas boiled, then strained, then {291} baked, and canned tomatoes. When fresh, I use the tomatoes uncooked with bread. This is my principal article of food." (FP—*Pamphlet 144, The Place of Herbs in Rational Therapy, 24; Selected Messages,* book 2, 294)

1897—*Medical Ministry*, 227–229.

"DRUG MEDICATION is to be discarded. On this point the conscience of the physician must ever be kept tender and true and clean. The inclination to use POISONOUS DRUGS, which kill if they do not cure, needs to be guarded against. Matters have been laid open before me in reference

to the use of DRUGS. Many have been {228} treated with DRUGS and the result has been death. Our physicians, by practicing DRUG MEDICA-TION, have lost many cases that need not have died if they had left their DRUGS out of the sickroom.
(*Pamphlet 144, The Place of Herbs in Rational Therapy,* 10)

"Fever cases have been lost, when, had the physicians left off entirely their DRUG treatment, had they put their wits to work and wisely and persistently used the Lord's own remedies, plenty of air and water, the patients would have recovered. The reckless use of these things that should be discarded has decided the case of the sick.

"Experimenting in DRUGS is a very expensive business. Paralysis of the brain and tongue is often the result, and the victims die an unnatural death, when, if they had been treated perseveringly, with unwearied, unrelaxed diligence with hot and cold water, hot compresses, packs, and dripping sheet, they would be alive today.
(*Pamphlet 144, The Place of Herbs in Rational Therapy,* 10–11)

"Nothing should be put into the human system that will leave a baleful influence behind. And to carry out the light on this subject, to practice hygienic treatment, is the reason which has been given me for establishing sanitariums in various localities.

"I have been pained when many students have been encouraged to go where they would receive an education in the use of DRUGS. The light I have received on the subject of DRUGS is altogether different from the use made of them at these schools or at the sanitariums. We must become enlightened on these subjects.

"The intricate names given MEDICINES are used to cover up the matter, so that none will know what is given them as remedies unless they consult a dictionary. . . .

"Patients are to be supplied with good, wholesome food; total abstinence from all INTOXICATING DRINKS is to be observed; DRUGS are to be discarded, and rational methods of treatment followed. The patients must not be given ALCOHOL, TEA, COFFEE, or DRUGS; for these always leave traces of evil behind them. By observing these rules, many who have been given up by the physicians may be restored to health.

"In this work the human and divine instrumentalities can cooperate in saving life, and God will add His blessing. Many suffering ones not of our faith will come to our institutions to {229} receive treatment. Those whose health has been ruined by sinful indulgence, and who have been treated by physicians till the DRUGS administered have no effect, will

Spirit of Prophecy References

come; and they will be benefited.

"The Lord will bless institutions conducted in accordance with His plans. He will cooperate with every physician who faithfully and conscientiously engages in this work. He will enter the rooms of the sick. He will give wisdom to the nurses."

1897—*Pamphlet 144, The Place of Herbs in Rational Therapy*, 10.

"Those who make a practice of taking DRUGS, sin against their intelligence and endanger their whole after life.

"There are HERBS that are harmless, the use of which will tide over many apparently serious difficulties."

1897—*Selected Messages*, book 2, 289–291.

"Your question is, . . . 'In urgent cases, should we call in a worldly physician, because the sanitarium doctors are all so busy that they have no time to devote to outside {290} practice?' If the physicians are so busy that they cannot treat the sick outside of the institution, would it not be wiser for all to educate themselves in the use of simple remedies, than to venture to use DRUGS that are given a long name to hide their real qualities. Why need anyone be ignorant of God's remedies—hot-water fomentations and cold and hot compresses. It is important to become familiar with the benefit of dieting in case of sickness. All should understand what to do [for] themselves. They may call upon someone who understands nursing, but everyone should have an intelligent knowledge of the house he lives in. All should understand what to do in case of sickness."
(*Manuscript Releases*, vol. 20, 1; *The Paulson Collection of Ellen G. White Letters*, 14)

"Were I sick, I would just as soon call in a lawyer as a physician from among general practitioners. (See Appendix A) I would not touch their NOSTRUMS, to which they give Latin names. I am determined to know, in straight English, the name of everything that I introduce into my system.
(*Pamphlet 144, The Place of Herbs in Rational Therapy*, 9–10; *Manuscript Releases*, vol. 20, 1; *The Paulson Collection of Ellen G. White Letters*, 14)

"Those who make a practice of taking DRUGS sin against {291} their intelligence and endanger their whole afterlife. There are HERBS that are harmless, the use of which will tide over many apparently serious difficulties. But if all would seek to become intelligent in regard to their bodily necessities, sickness would be rare instead of common. An

ounce of prevention is worth a pound of cure."
(*Manuscript Releases,* vol. 20, 1; *The Paulson Collection of Ellen G. White Letters,* 15)

1897—*Temperance,* 58.

"Intemperance of every kind is holding human beings as in a vise. TOBACCO inebriates are multiplying. What shall we say of this evil? It is unclean; it is a NARCOTIC; it stupefies the senses; it chains the will; it holds its victims in the slavery of habits difficult to overcome; it has Satan for its advocate. It destroys the clear perceptions of the mind that sin and corruption may not be distinguished from truth and holiness. This appetite for TOBACCO is self-destructive. It leads to a craving for something stronger—FERMENTED WINES and LIQUORS, all of which are intoxicating."

1897—*The Kress Collection,* 48.

"Those who have had privileges and opportunities and light upon light will find themselves brought into comparison with those whose religious advantages have been limited, and who have made diligent, persevering effort to lay hold of eternal life. Over such the Lord rejoiceth with singing. The whole heathen world will rise up in judgment against those whom Heaven has favored the most, but have placed themselves on Satan's side, and worked in his lines to bring their soul-destroying NARCOTICS to foreign lands, to pollute and destroy the heathen nations with their defiling and HEALTH-DE-STROYING DRUGS. For the sake of revenue, a professedly Christian nation have forced their traffic upon heathen nations at the point of the sword, and thus compel them to accept their merchandise, which would in using degrade the people below the level of the brute creation.
(*Manuscript Releases,* vol. 3, 341–342)

"Christ came to our world to restore the moral image of God in men; but the men who have had great light have given themselves over to Satan. They have worked out his plans in introducing TOBACCO, LIQUOR and OPIUM into foreign, heathen lands. And these things have been recognized by the intelligent heathen as a deadly evil that leads to all kinds of violence and crime, and stirs up the savage elements to delight in war. Thus ungovernable propensities are perpetuated, making it almost hopeless to send missionaries among them. And the heathen hate the white man for this kind of work."

Spirit of Prophecy References

1897—*The Paulson Collection of Ellen G. White Letters*, 14.

"Your letter to me, under date of February 12, is received. Your question is, 'Is it advisable to employ a good, Christian physician, who treats his patients on hygiene principles? In urgent cases, should we call in a worldly physician, because the Sanitarium doctors are all so busy that they have no time to devote to outside practice? Some say that when the Sanitarium doctors do use DRUGS, they give larger doses than ordinary doctors."
(*Manuscript Releases*, vol. 20, 1)

1898—*Spalding and Magan Collection*, 140.

"There is a work to be done by our churches that few have any idea of. 'I was an hungered,' Christ says, 'and ye gave me meat: I was thirsty, and ye gave me drink: I was a stranger, and ye took me in: naked, and ye clothed me: I was sick, and ye visited me: {23} I was in prison, and ye came unto me.' Matthew 25:35–36. We shall have to give of our means to support laborers in the harvest field, and we shall rejoice in the sheaves gathered in. But while this is right, there is a work as yet untouched that must be done. The mission of Christ was to heal the sick, encourage the hopeless, bind up the brokenhearted. This work of restoration is to be carried on among the needy, suffering ones of humanity. God calls not only for your benevolence, but your cheerful countenance, your hopeful words, the grasp of your hand. Relieve some of God's afflicted ones. Some are sick and hope has departed. Bring back the sunlight to them. There are souls who have lost their courage; speak to them, pray for them. There are those who need the Bread of Life. Read to them from the Word of God. There is a soul sickness no balm can reach, no MEDICINE heal. Pray for them, and bring them to Jesus Christ. And in all your work, Christ will be present to make impressions upon human hearts."
(*A Call to Medical Evangelism and Health Education*, 22–23;
LP—*The Health Food Ministry*, 42)

1898—*Counsels on Diet and Foods*, 293–294.

"I met the doctors and Brother——, and talked with them for about two hours, and I freed my soul. I told them that they had been tempted, and that they were yielding to temptation. In order to secure patronage, they would set a meat table, and then they would be tempted to go farther, to use TEA and COFFEE and DRUGS. . . . I said, There will be temptation through the ones whose appetite for meat has been gratified, and if such ones have connection with the Health Home, they will present temptations to sacrifice principle. There must not be the first introduction of meat eating. Then there will not need to be an expulsion of meat, because it will never have appeared on the table. . . . The argument had been used, that they might use meat upon the table until they could educate in regard to its disuse. But as new patients were continually coming, the same excuse would establish meat eating. No; do not let it appear {294} on the table once. Then your lectures in regard to the meat question will correspond with the message you should bear."

1898—*The Ellen G. White Biography,* 1891–1900, vol. 4, 356–357.

"We are to be sure that we commence the work in right lines. {357} No TEA, no COFFEE; avoid DRUGS. We are to take our position firmly in regard to the light given us that the consumption of the dead flesh of animals is counterworking the restoring of the sick to health. It is not a safe and wholesome diet. . . .'"

1898—*Manuscript Releases,* vol. 3, 367.

"The study of the Word is greatly neglected. If the Word is studied with humility of mind, the Holy Spirit will make its application. 'The entrance of Thy words giveth light,' says the psalmist. 'It giveth understanding unto the simple.' Psalms 119:130. It sends forth to all who study its divine principles precious beams of light. It is better than ANY DRUGS, and will give physical soundness."

1898—*Manuscript Releases,* vol. 4, 97.

"Men are dealing in LIQUORS and NARCOTICS that are destroying the human family. DEATHLY MIXTURES are used that make men mad, and murder and violence are prevailing everywhere."

1898—*Medical Ministry,* 235.

"Therefore personal religion for all physicians in the sickroom is essential to success in giving the simple treatment without DRUGS. He who is a physician and guardian of the health and body, God would have in every way educated to learn lessons of the Great Teacher how to work in Christ and through Christ to save the souls of the sick. How can any physician know this until the Saviour shall be received as a personal Saviour to him who administers to suffering humanity?"

1898—*Mind, Character, and Personality,* vol. 2, 407.

"The Lord would have our minds clear and sharp, able to see points in His Word and service, doing His will, depending upon His grace,

bringing into His work a clear conscience and a thankful mind. This kind of joy promotes the circulation of the blood. Vital energy is imparted to the mind through the brain; therefore the brain should never be dulled by the use of NARCOTICS or excited by the use of STIMULANTS. Brain, bone, and muscle are to be brought into harmonious action that all may work as well-regulated machines, each part acting in harmony, not one being overtaxed."
(LP—*Temperance*, 74)

1898—*Pamphlet 144, The Place of Herbs in Rational Therapy*, 11–12.

"Nothing should be put into the human system that will leave a baleful influence behind. And to carry out the light on this subject, to practice hygienic treatment, is the reason which has been given me for establishing sanitariums in various localities. . . .

"We must become enlightened on these subjects. The intricate names given MEDICINE are used to cover up the matter, so that none will know what is given them as remedies unless they consult a dictionary. . . . {12}

"It is a delusion and a farce, and the Lord has revealed to me that this practice would not preserve life, but would introduce into the system those things which should never be there, for they would do a deleterious work on the human organism."

1898—*Spalding and Magan Collection*, 137.

"Many physicians in our world are of no benefit to the human family. The DRUG SCIENCE has been exalted, but if every bottle that comes from every such institution were done away with, there would be fewer invalids in the world today. DRUG MEDICATION should never have been introduced into our institutions. There was no need of this being so, and for this very reason the LORD would have us establish an institution where He can come in and where His grace and power can be revealed. 'I am the resurrection and the life,' (John 11:25) He declares.
(*Pamphlet 144, The Place of Herbs in Rational Therapy*, 12)

"The true method for healing the sick is to tell them of the HERBS that grow for the benefit of man. Scientists have attached large names to these simplest preparations, but true education will lead us to teach the sick that they need not call in a doctor any more than they would call in a lawyer. They can themselves administer the SIMPLE HERBS if necessary. To educate the human family that the doctor alone knows all the ills of infants and persons of every age, is false teaching, and the sooner

we as a people stand on the principles of health reform, the greater will be the blessing that will come to those who would do true medical work. There is a work to be done in treating the sick with water and teaching them to make the most of sunshine and physical exercise. Thus in simple language we may teach the people how to preserve health, how to avoid sickness. This is the work our sanitariums are called upon to do. This is true science."
(*Pamphlet 144, The Place of Herbs in Rational Therapy,* 13)

1898—*Spalding and Magan Collection,* 140–141.

"To a large extent Satan has carried out his plans. The Lord's property is embezzled; God is robbed. The means that has been lent to man to relieve the necessities of the poor and to uplift and sustain the fallen in righteousness and truth, is used to please and {141} glorify self. From the beginning to the end the crime of TOBACCO USING, of OPIUM and DRUG MEDICATION, has its origin in perverted knowledge. It is through plucking and eating of POISONOUS FRUIT, through the intricacies of names that the common people do not understand, that thousands and ten thousands of lives are lost. This great knowledge, supposed by man to be so wonderful, God did not mean that man should have. They are using the POISONOUS PRODUCTIONS that Satan himself has planted to take the place of the tree of life, whose leaves are for the healing of the nations. Men are dealing in LIQUORS and NARCOTICS that are destroying the human family. DEATHLY MIXTURES are used, that make men mad, and murder and violence are prevailing everywhere."
(MP—*Temperance,* 75)

1898—*The Desire of Ages,* 824.

"In the Saviour's manner of healing there were lessons for His disciples. On one occasion He anointed the eyes of a blind man with CLAY, and bade him, 'Go, wash in the pool of Siloam. . . . He went his way therefore, and washed, and came seeing.' John 9:7. The cure could be wrought only by the power of the Great Healer, yet Christ made use of the simple agencies of nature. While He did not give countenance to DRUG MEDICATION, He sanctioned the use of simple and natural remedies."
(*Counsels on Health,* 30; *Gospel Workers,* 221; *The Ministry of Healing,* 233; *Testimony Studies on Diet and Foods,* 85)

1898—*The Paulson Collection of Ellen G. White Letters,* 31.

"As to DRUGS being used in our institutions, it is contrary to the light which the Lord has been pleased to give. The DRUGGING BUSINESS has done more harm to our world and killed more than it has helped or cured. The light was first given to me why institutions should be established, that is, sanitariums were to reform the medical practices of physicians. This is God's method. The HERBS that grow for the benefit of man, and the little HANDFUL of HERBS kept and steeped for sudden ailments, have served tenfold, yes, one hundred-fold better purpose, than all the DRUGS hidden under mysterious names and dealt out to the sick. It is a delusion and farce, and the Lord has revealed to me that this practice would not preserve life, but would introduce into the system those things which should never be there, for they would do a deleterious work on the human organism.

(FP—*Pamphlet 144, The Place of Herbs in Rational Therapy,* 12; *Medical Ministry,* 27)

"The living connection with the Great Physician is worth more than connection with a world of DRUGS. The soothing power of pure truth, seen, and maintained in all its bearings, is of a value no language can express, to people who are suffering with disease.

Keep ever before the suffering sick the compassion and tenderness of Christ, and awaken their conscience to a belief in His power to relieve suffering, and lead them to faith and trust in Him, the Great Healer, and you have gained a soul and oftentimes a life.

(*Testimony Studies on Diet and Foods,* 85)

"Therefore, personal religion for all physicians in the sickroom is essential to success in giving the simple treatments without DRUGS. He who is a physician and guardian of the health and body, God would have everyone educated to learn lessons of the Great Teacher, how to work in Christ and through Christ to save the souls of the sick. How can any physician know this until the Saviour shall be received as a personal Saviour to him who administers to suffering humanity?"

1898—*The Use of Drugs in the Care of the Sick*, Ellen G. White Publications Manuscript, 24.

"We should not use the DRUGS and NARCOTICS used by worldly physicians to relieve the necessity which the abuse of appetite has created in the physical structure."

1898—*The Use of Drugs in the Care of the Sick*, Ellen G. White Publications Manuscript, 36.

"The ambassadors of Christ can be doubly useful if they know how to restore the diseased to health. This was the work of Christ. But as in prayer we present these suffering ones to the Lord for His healing power to come to them, the people themselves must be instructed to do those things which will assist nature, not in DRUG MEDICATION, but in the use of the agencies the Lord has prepared—sunlight, pure air, pure water, healthful exercise. These things possess a power which millions in our world know nothing of. These restoring agencies must be used intelligently, and as we do all that it is in our power to do, we must mingle with our work our earnest prayers."

1898—*The Paulson Collection of Ellen G. White Letters*, 47–48.

"But instead of cooperating with the mighty Healer, by using the very means He has provided, by educating themselves to use water and fresh air, and to avoid all uncleanness of person and premises, they turn to physicians who are in no way connected with the Lord Jesus, and take their PRESCRIPTIONS of DRUG MEDICATIONS. These leave their POISONOUS TRAIL behind, implanting in the system seeds of suffering and death. Why do they not inquire of God? Why do they not seek help from the One who so loved them that He gave His only begotten Son to save all who would believe on Him? Is He not just as well able now to heal disease as when He walked in humanity upon the earth? Where is our faith when we turn to every conceivable resource but to the One who declares that He came to the world to do a special work in healing the sick. Why are not all who accept Christ so illuminated that they can irradiate others, and lift them from grovelling in intemperance of all kinds, leading them to let DRUGS alone. . . . {48}

"The Lord will heal those who believe, but He has given natural blessings for the benefit of the afflicted, and He would have these used. God could have healed Hezekiah with a word. But He heard Hezekiah's prayer, and gave directions that a bunch of FIGS be placed upon the diseased parts. This was done, and Hezekiah recovered. But his recovery was not instantaneous. He had not the same faith that the afflicted woman had. We need to exercise faith. To practice the use of DRUG MEDICATION does not harmonize with faith. Appealing to worldly physicians is dishonoring to God. Those who come to God in faith must cooperate with Him in accepting and using His Heaven-sent remedies—water, sunlight, and plenty of air."

Spirit of Prophecy References

1899—*The Ellen G. White Biography*, 1891–1900, vol. 4, 437.

"Sister McEnterfer is nurse and physician for all the region round about. She has been called upon to treat the most difficult cases, and with complete success. We have at times made our house a hospital, where we have taken in the sick and cared for them. I have not time to relate the wonderful cures wrought, not by the dosing with DRUGS, but by the application of water."

1899—*Battle Creek Letters*, 15–16.

"The Lord has connected Dr. Kellogg with the medical fraternity outside our people. His influence has had much to do with the abolishing of DRUGS to a large extent, and the introduction of nature's own restoratives. This work has not been done by making a raid upon DRUGS, for it needed the wisdom of a serpent and the harmlessness of a dove. Dr. Kellogg's connection with {16} God enables him to take the presence of the Holy Spirit with him into assemblies where there is generally much levity, and where many things are spoken that might better be left unsaid. The people respect the doctor's religious principles, and show that they are somewhat under the influence of this faith."

1899—*The Ellen G. White Biography*, 1900–1905, vol. 5, 284.

"The air is God's MEDICINE, and good food is God's MEDICINE. There is power, life, in the pure water, because God's life is in it."

1899—*Evangelism*, 529.

"Satan is taking the world captive through the use of LIQUOR and TOBACCO, TEA and COFFEE. The God-given mind, which should be kept clear, is perverted by the use of NARCOTICS. The brain is no longer able to distinguish correctly. The enemy has control. Man has sold his reason for that which makes him mad. He has no sense of what is right. Yet the LIQUOR CURSE is legalized, and works untold ruin in the hands of those who love to tamper with that which not only ruins the poor victim but his whole family.
(*Temperance*, 17)

"The curse of LIQUOR DRINKING is demonstrated by the awful murders that take place. Intemperance is widespread. How much man's senses are perverted by INTOXICATING DRUGS it is impossible to say."

1899—*Review and Herald,* April 18, 1899.

"On the evening after the third Sabbath, Dr. Caro spoke to nearly three thousand persons on the subject, 'The Man and the Habit.' The lecture was illustrated by limelight views showing the terrible power of habit as seen in the downward course of the drunkard, from the innocent child to the sin-hardened criminal. Solemn and instructive was this object lesson. The effects of the TOBACCO CURSE, the LIQUOR CURSE, the OPIUM CURSE, were vividly portrayed. Then a powerful appeal was made for the shielding of the youth from evil associations, and for the offer of a helping hand to the tempted and the fallen. At the close, several hymns—'God Be With You Till We Meet Again,' and others—were shown on the screen, and sung by the whole audience, with an earnestness and feeling that made my heart glad."

1899—*Manuscript Releases,* vol. 1, 66.

"The Lord gave me special light in regard to the establishment of a health reform institution, where treatment of the sick could be carried on on altogether different lines from those existing in any institution in our world. It must be founded and conducted on Bible principles, and be the Lord's instrumentality, not to cure with DRUGS, but to use Nature's remedies. Those who have any connection with this institution must be educated in health-restoring principles."
(*Manuscript Releases,* vol. 20, 249)

1899—*Manuscript Releases,* vol. 4, 98.

"The Lord gave men minds in order that He might control them. But Satan has come in with a determination to control the minds of men. . . . He has led men into . . . the use of the NARCOTIC TOBACCO, of OPIUM, and all other DRUGS which weaken the hold of the human family upon life."

1899—*Manuscript Releases,* vol. 11, 98.

"Never was there a place where medical missionary work would have told with more power than in Australia. But in our efforts to do this work we have been handicapped for want of means. The money we should have had to invest in a sanitarium has been used in erecting sanitariums in places where they were not so much needed. The Lord Jesus Christ was the greatest Physician this world has ever known. We cannot in the full sense of the word call Him a medical missionary. He was the Divine Healer. He was imbued with power to heal all manner of diseases without resorting to DRUGS."

Spirit of Prophecy References

1899—*Review and Herald,* June 27, 1899.

"The souls as well as the bodies of the youth are affected by the habits of eating and drinking. Wrong habits render the youth less susceptible to Bible instruction. God calls upon parents to guard their children against the indulgence of appetite, and especially against the use of STIMULANTS and NARCOTICS. The tables of Christian parents should never be loaded down with food containing condiments and spices. They are to study to preserve the stomach from any abuse. Fathers and mothers may do much in giving right characters to their children by controlling their own appetites and passions. Fathers who use TOBACCO and LIQUOR POISON their blood, and transmit to their children their own vitiated habits intensified. They give them as a legacy feeble moral powers. Thus the sins of parents are perpetuated in their offspring. In the day of final account, what a weight of crime will be charged to parents who have neglected their duty to themselves and their children."
(*Child Guidance,* 405)

1899—*Manuscript Releases,* vol. 16, 247.

"There is to be a sanitarium in Australia, and altogether new methods of treating the sick are to be practiced. DRUG MEDICATION must be left out of the question if the human physician would receive the diploma written and issued in heaven. There are many physicians who will never receive this diploma unless they learn in the school of the Great Physician. This means that they must unlearn and cast away the supposed wonderful knowledge of how to treat disease with POISONOUS DRUGS. They must go to God's great laboratory of nature, and there learn the simplest methods of using the remedies which the Lord has furnished. When DRUGS are thrown aside, when FERMENTED LIQUOR of all kinds is discarded, when God's remedies—sunshine, pure air, water, and good food—are used, there will be far fewer deaths and a far greater number of cures."

1899—*Selected Messages,* book 2, 288–289.

"Christ never planted the seeds of death in the system. Satan planted these seeds when he tempted Adam to eat of the tree of knowledge which meant disobedience to God. Not one NOXIOUS PLANT was placed in the Lord's great garden, but after Adam and Eve sinned, POISONOUS HERBS sprang up. In the parable of the sower the question was asked the master, 'Didst not thou sow good seed in thy field? from whence then hath it tares?' The master answered, 'An enemy hath done this.'

Matthew 13:27–28. All tares are sown by the evil one. Every NOXIOUS HERB is of his sowing, and by his ingenious methods of amalgamation he has corrupted the earth with tares.
(*Manuscript Releases,* vol. 16, 247;
LP—*S.D.A. Bible Commentary,* vol.1, 1086)

"Then shall physicians continue to resort to DRUGS, which leave a deadly evil in the system, destroying that life which {289} Christ came to restore? Christ's remedies cleanse the system. But Satan has tempted man to introduce into the system that which weakens the human machinery, clogging and destroying the fine, beautiful arrangements of God. The DRUGS administered to the sick do not restore, but destroy. DRUGS never cure. Instead, they place in the system seeds which bear a very bitter harvest. . . .
(*Pamphlet 144, The Place of Herbs in Rational Therapy,* 14; *Manuscript Releases,* vol. 16, 247–248)

"Our Saviour is the restorer of the moral image of God in man. He has supplied in the natural world remedies for the ills of man, that His followers may have life and that they may have it more abundantly. We can with safety discard the CONCOCTIONS which man has used in the past. (See Appendix A)
(*Pamphlet 144, The Place of Herbs in Rational Therapy,* 14; *Manuscript Releases,* vol. 16, 248)

"The Lord has provided antidotes for diseases in SIMPLE PLANTS, (see Appendix A) and these can be used by faith, with no denial of faith; for by using the blessings provided by God for our benefit we are cooperating with Him. He can use water and sunshine and the HERBS which He has caused to grow, in healing maladies brought on by indiscretion or accident. We do not manifest a lack of faith when we ask God to bless His remedies. True faith will thank God for the knowledge of how to use these precious blessings in a way which will restore mental and physical vigor. The body is to be carefully cared for, and in this the Lord demands the cooperation of the human agent. Man must become intelligent in regard to the treatment and use of brain, bone, and muscle. The very best experience we can gain is to know ourselves."
(*Manuscript Releases,* vol. 16, 248–249)

1899—*Manuscript Releases,* vol. 16, 287–290.

"The influence you have gained in the medical profession is large and broad, and in some respects it has been as God would have it. You have {288} caused the light God has given you to shine forth to others, and this light has influenced others to labor in the different lines of the medical work. But according to the light the Lord has given me, something of the spirit of Freemasonry (See Appendix A) exists, and has built a wall about the work. The old, regular practice has been exalted as the only true method for the treatment of disease. And to a large degree this feeling has leavened the physicians connected with you. They have resorted to DRUGS in cases of fever—to break it up, as they have thought. This method has broken up fevers and other diseases, but in some cases it has broken up the whole man with it.

"The Lord has been pleased to present this matter before me in clear lines. Fever cases need not be treated with DRUGS. The most difficult cases are best and most successfully managed by nature's own resources. This science, fully adopted, will bring the best results, if the practitioner will be thorough. The Lord will bless the physician who depends on natural methods, helping every function of the human machinery to act in its own strength the part the Lord designed it to act in restoring itself to proper action.

"Dr. Kellogg, God has given you favor with the medical fraternity, and he would have you hold that favor. But in no case are you to stand as do the physicians of the world to exalt allopathy above every other practice, and call all other methods quackery and error; for from the beginning to the present time the results of allopathy have made a most objectionable {289} showing. There has been loss of life in your sanitarium because DRUGS have been administered, and these give no chance for nature to do her work of restoration. DRUG MEDICATION has broken up the power of the human machinery, and the patients have died. Others have carried the DRUGS away with them, making less effective the simple remedies nature uses to restore the system. The students in your institution [Battle Creek Sanitarium] are not to be educated to regard DRUGS as a necessity. They are to be educated to leave DRUGS alone.
(*Manuscript Releases,* vol. 3, 305)

"The medical fraternity, represented to me as Freemasonry, with their long, unintelligible names which common people cannot understand, would call the Lord's prescription for Hezekiah quackery. Death was pronounced upon the king, but he prayed for life, and his prayer was heard. Those who had the care of him were told to get a bunch of FIGS and put them on the sore, and the king was restored. This means was taken by God to teach them that all their preparations were only depriving the king of the power to rally and overcome disease. While they pursued their course of treatment, his life could not be saved. The Lord diverted their minds from their wonderful mysteries to a simple remedy of nature.

"There are lessons for us all in these directions. Young men who are sent to Ann Arbor to obtain an education which they think will exalt them as supreme in their treatment of disease by DRUGS, will find that it will result in the loss of life rather than restoration to health and strength. These MIXTURES place a double taxation upon nature, and in the effort to {290} throw off the POISONS they contain, thousands of persons lose their lives. We must leave DRUGS entirely alone, for in using them we introduce an enemy into the system. I write this because we have to meet this DRUG MEDICATION in the physicians in this country, and we do not want this practice, as in Battle Creek, to steal into our midst as a thief. We want the door closed against the enemy before the lives of human beings are imperiled."

1899—*(Australasian) Union Conference Record,* July 28, 1899.

"When God's people show that they realize their accountability to Him, and their dependence on Him, by carrying forward His work, the Lord blesses them. We are to do the very best we can. We must have a Sanitarium, and we must have it out of the city, in a convenient location, where there is plenty of water, because we use water in the place of DRUGS. The Sanitarium is to be located in a restful place, where trams are not passing all the time. It should be away from the smoke of the chimneys of a city, where the atmosphere is as pure as can be found. We can be in touch with Sydney, and yet be out of Sydney. Christ prayed for His people. 'I pray not that thou shouldst take them out of the world, but that thou shouldst keep them from the evil.' John 17:15. We are not to leave the world, but we are to avoid all the evil possible. The Lord God of Israel is going to help us in this matter, and we are going to seek Him with heart and soul. We are going to plead that God will let His Holy Spirit rest upon us. He will hearken to the testimony of faith, and I believe we shall see the salvation of God. I believe He will furnish good counselors, men who can think in right lines, and He will work with them. I have no confidence in the smartest men that ever lived unless they are under the control of God. They may have natural capabilities and talents, but unless they are guided by the Holy Spirit, they will be controlled by someone else. God has given us talents, and He wants us to place ourselves under His working power. And just as sure as we do this, He will give us power to work."

Spirit of Prophecy References

1899—*Manuscript Releases*, vol. 17, 139.

"The coal mines must have the truth brought to them. The suburbs must be worked. A hospital must be built in Cooranbong. Dr. Kellogg assures me that he will raise $1,000 for this. We shall get believers and unbelievers to donate labor to clear the one acre of land on which the house is to be built. One man has promised to give the logs for building. We are suffering for [the lack of} this building for our sick. One man was taken sick. When the doctor came he did not put his hand upon him, [only] left a little MEDICINE, and charged two guineas. It is just terrible. The doctors do scarcely anything for the sick. Dr. Rand came and found that the man had had no action of the bladder for days and no movement of the bowels for more than a week. The doctor from Newcastle had asked nothing about his condition."

1899—*Medical Ministry*, 125.

"It is time for the people of God, those who wear the sign of His kingdom, and whose authority is derived from 'It is written,' to work. The world is the field of our labor, and we are to strive to give the last message of mercy to the world. Our every action is being watched with jealous eyes. Be on guard as physicians. You can serve the Lord in your position by working with new methods and discarding DRUGS." (*Manuscript Releases*, vol. 15, 39)

1899—*Manuscript Releases*, vol. 21, 41–42.

"The fact that Christ when He was on this earth was a Healer of all manner of disease, is an encouragement and hope amid the moral sickness and evil that prevails; and we should do far more as physicians and nurses, as ministers of righteousness, if, instead of looking down into the grave, we fixed our gaze upon the mighty Healer. Whatever the disorder may be, the glories of the heavenly will do more for the saving of body and soul than all the DRUG MEDICATION in the world, than all the terrors of the grave will do if kept before the helpless and apparently hopeless. . . .

"You need, my brother, to place burdens and responsibilities upon others, while you preside. You can be worked by the Holy Spirit to devise and plan after the order of God. But trust not to your own human wisdom. Trust not to POISONOUS DRUGS that will interfere with nature's work and leave their cruel trail behind. Work away from DRUGS, and never, never advise one under your influence to go to Ann Arbor or any other place to obtain the education supposed to be essential for the perfection of the medical practitioner. The stamp left upon them by such places is almost ineffaceable. Educate, educate, educate, by placing yourself and others in the closest connection with the greatest Healer the world has ever known. Keep in view the better world, which is attracting to itself all {42} who are receiving the grace of God in this world."

1899—*Review and Herald,* September 5, 1899.

"In such cases the sufferers can do for themselves that which others cannot do as well for them. They should begin to relieve nature of the load they have forced upon her. They should remove the cause by fasting a short time, and giving the stomach time to rest. The feverish state of the system should be reduced by a careful and understanding application of water. These efforts will help nature in her struggle to free the system of impurities. But generally the persons who suffer pain become impatient. They are not willing to practice self-denial, and suffer a little from hunger, neither are they willing to wait the slow process of nature to build up the overtaxed energies of the system; but they are determined to obtain relief at once, and so take POWERFUL DRUGS, prescribed by physicians. Nature was doing her work well, and would have triumphed; but while accomplishing her task, a FOREIGN SUBSTANCE of a POISONOUS NATURE was introduced. What a mistake! Abused nature has now two evils to war against instead of one. She leaves the work in which she was engaged, and resolutely takes hold to expel the intruder newly introduced into the system. Nature feels this double draft upon her resources, and becomes enfeebled."

1899—*The Paulson Collection of Ellen G. White Letters,* 26–27.

"I have some things to say to you which you need. There are places you might fill, places in which you might be a blessing in many ways. But erroneous ideas keep you from filling these places. Your character needs to be pruned; for there is a superfluous growth that needs to be cut away from you. The idea which you hold that no REMEDIES should be used for the sick is an error. God does not heal the sick without the aid of the means of healing which lie within the reach of man; or when men refuse to be benefited by the SIMPLE REMEDIES that God has provided in pure air and water.

(LP—*Selected Messages,* book 2, 286)

"There were physicians in Christ's day and in the days of the apostles. Luke is called the beloved physician. He trusted in the Lord to make him skillful in the application of remedies. When the Lord told Hezekiah that He would spare his life for fifteen years, and as a sign that He would fulfill His promise, caused the sun to go back ten degrees, why did He not put His direct, restoring power upon the king? He told him to apply a BUNCH of FIGS to his sore, and that natural remedy blessed by God, healed him. The God of nature directs the human agent to use natural remedies now.

(*Selected Messages,* book 2, 286–287;
LP—*Pamphlet 144, The Place of Herbs in Rational Therapy,* 16–17)

"I might go to any length in this matter, my brother, but I leave it now with a few instances. A brother was taken sick with inflammation of the {27} bowels and bloody dysentery. The man was not a careful health reformer, but indulged his appetite. We were just preparing to leave Texas, where we had been laboring for several months, and we had carriages prepared to take away this brother and his family, and several others who were suffering from malarial fever. My husband and I thought we would stand this expense rather than have the heads of several families die and leave their wives and children unprovided for. Two or three were taken in a spring wagon on spring mattresses. But this man who was suffering from inflammation of the bowels, sent for me to come to him. My husband and I decided that it would not do to move him. Fears were entertained that mortification had set in. Then the thought came to me like a communication from the Lord, to take PULVERIZED CHARCOAL, put water upon it, and give this water to the sick man to drink, putting bandages of the CHARCOAL over the bowels and stomach. We were about one mile from the city of Dennison, but the sick man's son went to a blacksmith's shop, secured the CHARCOAL, and pulverized it, and then used it according to the directions given. The result was that in half an hour there was a change for the better. We had to go on our journey and leave the family behind, but what was our surprise the following day to see their wagon overtake us. The sick man was lying in a bed in the wagon. The blessing of God had worked with the simple means used."

(FP—*Selected Messages,* book 2, 287;
LP— *Selected Messages,* book 2, 299; *Pamphlet 144, The Place of Herbs in Rational Therapy,* 22–23)

"I still remember another case. At our first camp meeting here, held in Brighton, a young lady was taken sick on the ground, and remained sick during most of the meeting. She was thought to have typhoid fever, and although many prayers were offered in her behalf, she left the ground sick.

Spirit of Prophecy References

Dr. M. C. Kellogg, half-brother to J. H. Kellogg, of Battle Creek, was attending her. He came to me one morning, and said, Sister Price is in great pain. I cannot relieve her. She cannot sleep, and every breath seems as though it would be her last. We prayed for her, and then like a flash of lightning there came to me the thought of the charcoal. 'Send to the blacksmith for CHARCOAL, and pulverize it,' I said, 'and put a poultice of it on her side.' He tried this, and in one hour he came to me and said, 'That prescription was an inspiration from God. Sister Price could not have lived until now if no change had come.' The sick one fell into a restful sleep; the crisis passed, and she began to amend. In a few days she was taken from Melbourne to her home in _____, and is alive and well today.

"All these things teach us that we are to be very careful lest we receive radical ideas and impressions. Your ideas regarding DRUG MEDICATION, I must respect; but even in this you must not always let the patients know that you discard DRUGS entirely until they become intelligent on the subject. You often place yourself in positions where you hurt your influence and do no one any good, by expressing all your convictions. Thus you cut yourself away from the people. You should modify your strong prejudice."
(*Selected Messages,* book 2, 287)

1899—*Temperance,* 261–262.

"I speak most decidedly on this subject [temperance], and it has a telling influence upon other minds. Often the testimony is borne, 'I have not used ANY TOBACCO, WINE, or ANY STIMULANT or NARCOTIC since that discourse you gave upon temperance.' Now, they say, 'I must furnish myself with enlightened principles for action; for I want others to know the benefits I have received. This reformation involves great consequences to me and all with whom I come in contact. I will choose the better part, to work with Christ {262} with settled principles and aims, to win a crown of life as an overcomer.' "
(*Manuscript Releases,* vol. 7, 161)

1899—*Welfare Ministry,* 335.

"Now news has come to us that our beloved brother has come down with typhoid fever. Mr. Pringle is the only man in the village who knows anything about giving treatment without DRUGS; but six weeks ago he was called upon to attend Mr. B., who was also down with typhoid. He has stayed with him night and day, and has now returned to his home, worn out with the strain. So he cannot be depended on to nurse Brother C."

1899—*Review and Herald,* December 5, 1899.

"In no case should sick persons be deprived of a full supply of fresh air in pleasant weather. Their rooms may not always be so constructed as to allow the windows or doors to be opened without the draft coming directly upon them, thus exposing them to the taking of cold. In such cases windows and doors should be opened in an adjoining room, thus letting fresh air enter the room occupied by the sick. Fresh air will prove far more beneficial to sick persons than MEDICINE, and is far more essential to them than their food. They will do better and will recover sooner when deprived of food than when deprived of fresh air."

18??—*Pamphlet 66, Health, Philanthropic, and Medical Missionary Work,* 40–41.

"Physicians should be ambassadors for Christ in their specific work, and instead of giving {41} prominence to a special THEORY of MEDICINE which they advocate, by a godly life and conversation they should make prominent the fact that they are Christians. Not one of the SCHOOLS of MEDICINE highly lauded in the world is approved in the courts above, nor do they bear the heavenly superscription and endorsement. You are not justified in advocating one school above the others, as though it were the only one worthy of respect. Those who vindicate one SCHOOL of MEDICINE and bitterly condemn another are actuated by a zeal that is not according to knowledge. With what pharisaic pride some men look down upon others who have not received a diploma from the so-called standard school. All this proves that they cannot see afar off, and have not been purged from their old sins. They need to humble themselves at the cross of Calvary. This spirit will never be acknowledged in heaven, nor will men who cherish it hear the 'Well done.' Matthew 25:21. Some have been as zealous in exalting what their particular school advocated as though the Lord had specified that that method was the only one to be allowed. The use of DRUGS has resulted in far more harm than good; and should our physicians who claim to believe the truth almost entirely dispense with MEDICINE, and faithfully practice along the lines of the principles of hygiene, using nature's remedies, far greater success would attend their efforts."

Spirit of Prophecy References

18??—*Pamphlet 98, Testimony for the Church at Olcott, N. Y.,* 2–3.

"Sr. Lamson loves this world. She is naturally selfish. She has suffered much with bodily infirmities. God has permitted this affliction to come upon Sr. Lamson, and yet would not permit Satan to take her life. God designed through the furnace of affliction to loosen her grasp upon earthly treasures. Through suffering alone could this be done. Sr. Lamson is one of that class whose system has been poisoned by DRUGS. She ignorantly, has made herself what she is, by taking DRUGS; yet God did not suffer her life to be taken. He has lengthened her years of probation and {3} suffering that she might become sanctified through the truth, be purified, made white and tried, and through the furnace of affliction, lose her dross, and become more precious than fine gold, even than the golden wedge of Ophir. Love of the world has become so deeply rooted in the hearts of this brother and sister that it will require a severe trial to remove it."

18??—*Pamphlet 144, The Place of Herbs in Rational Therapy,* 29.

"You are not justified in advocating one school above the others as if it were the only one worthy of respect. Those who vindicate one SCHOOL of MEDICINE and bitterly condemn another, are actuated by a zeal that is not according to knowledge. With pharisaic pride some men look down upon others who have received a diploma from the so-called standard school. . . . The use of DRUGS has resulted in far more harm than good, and should our physicians who claim to believe the truth, almost entirely dispense with MEDICINE, and faithfully practice along the line of hygiene, using nature's remedies, far greater success would attend their efforts. There is no need whatever to exalt the method whereby DRUGS are administered. I know whereof I speak. Brethren of the medical profession, I entreat you to think candidly and put away childish things. . . . They resort to DRUGS when greater skill and knowledge would teach them the more excellent way."

1900—*Sanitarium Announcement,* January 1, 1900.

"Time is passing, and the work to be accomplished by our Sanitarium is as yet scarcely begun. In our institution we wish to teach health and temperance principles from the Bible standpoint. All need to understand how to preserve physical health, that the bodies which God has created may be presented to Him a living sacrifice, fitted to render Him acceptable service. The right balance of the mental and moral powers depends to a great degree upon the right condition and action of the physical system. Through indulgence of perverted appetite man loses his power to resist temptation. The sure effect of NARCOTICS and unnatural STIMULANTS as TEA, COFFEE, TOBACCO, BEER and WINE, is to enfeeble and degrade the physical nature, and lower the tone of intellect and morals. Any unnatural excitement of the nervous system affects the brain nerve power. We have a work before us to educate the people, line upon line, and precept upon precept. We must teach them that health and even life is endangered by the use of STIMULANTS which excite the exhausted energies to unnatural, spasmodic action.

"The people must be educated to understand that it is a sin to destroy their physical, mental, and spiritual energies. And they must understand how to cooperate with God in their own restoration. Through faith in Christ they can overcome the habit of using HEALTH-DESTROYING STIMULANTS and NARCOTICS."
(*Temperance*, 89)

1900—*The Signs of the Times*, March 14, 1900.

"Every student should understand how to take care of himself so as to preserve the best possible condition of health, resisting feebleness and disease; if from any cause disease does come, or accidents do occur, he should know how to meet ordinary emergencies without calling upon a physician and taking his POISONOUS DRUGS."
(*Special Testimonies on Education*, 34; *Fundamentals of Christian Education*, 426–427)

1900—*Testimonies*, vol. 6, 227–228.

"Wonderful is the work which God designs to accomplish through His servants, that His name may be glorified. God made Joseph a fountain of life to the Egyptian nation. Through Joseph the life of that whole people was preserved. Through Daniel God saved the life of all the wise men of Babylon. And these deliverances were as object lessons; they illustrated to the people the spiritual blessings offered them through connection with the God whom Joseph and Daniel worshiped. So through His people today God desires to bring blessings to the world. Every worker in whose heart Christ abides, everyone who will show forth His love to the world, is a worker together with God for the blessing of humanity. As he receives from the Saviour grace to impart to others, from his whole being flows forth the tide of spiritual life. Christ came as the Great Physician to heal the wounds that sin has made in the human family, and His Spirit, working through His servants,

Spirit of Prophecy References

imparts to sin-sick, suffering human beings a mighty healing power that is efficacious for the body and the soul. 'In that day,' says the Scriptures, 'there shall be a fountain opened to the house of David and to the inhabitants of Jerusalem for sin and for uncleanness.' Zechariah 13:1. The waters of this fountain contain MEDICINAL PROPERTIES that will heal both physical and spiritual infirmities.
(*Counsels on Health,* 209)

"From this fountain flows the mighty river seen in Ezekiel's vision. 'These waters issue out toward the east country, and go down into the desert, and go into the sea: which being brought forth into the sea, the waters shall {228} be healed. And it shall come to pass, that every thing that liveth, which moveth, whithersoever the rivers shall come, shall live. . . . And by the river upon the bank thereof, on this side and on that side, shall grow all trees for meat, whose leaf shall not fade, neither shall the fruit thereof be consumed: it shall bring forth new fruit according to his months, because their waters they issued out of the sanctuary: and the fruit thereof shall be for meat, and the leaf thereof for MEDICINE.' Ezekiel 47:8–9, 12."
(*Counsels on Health,* 210)

1900—*Review and Herald,* May 1, 1900.

"Christ prayed for his disciples and for us, 'As thou has sent me into the world, even so have I also sent them into the world.' 'Sanctify them through thy truth: thy word is truth.' John 17:18, 17. We have need of all the spiritual help that we can obtain in order to do the work to be done in this world. Satan is taking the world captive through the use of TEA and COFFEE, LIQUOR, and TOBACCO. The mind is dulled by the use of NARCOTICS. Can anyone make an impression on a man who is drunk? A drunken man is unable to distinguish between right and wrong, because the enemy has control of his brain. He has sold his reason for that which makes him mad. He has no sense of what is right; for the LIQUOR he drinks is so DRUGGED that it makes him insane. Satan spreads a net for his feet by tempting him to take the LIQUOR POISON, and he knows no more what he is doing than a madman."

1900—*Testimonies,* vol. 6, 302.

"Those who understand physiology and hygiene will, in their ministerial labor, find it a means whereby they may enlighten others in regard to the proper and intelligent treatment of the physical, mental, and moral powers. Therefore those who are preparing for the ministry should make

a diligent study of the human organism, that they may know how to care for the body, not by means of DRUGS, but from nature's own laboratory. The Lord will bless those who make every effort to keep themselves free from disease and lead others to regard as sacred the health of the body as well as of the soul."
(*Review and Herald,* January 14, 1902)

1900—*The Kress Collection,* 85–87.

"In the Sanitarium which we are about to erect in New South Wales, provision must be made for all classes. The accommodation and treatment must be such that patients of the higher class will be attracted to the institution. Rooms must be fitted for the use of those who are willing to pay a liberal price. Rational methods of treatment must be followed. The patients must not be given ALCOHOL, TEA, COFFEE, or DRUGS; for these always leave traces of evil behind. . . . {86}
(*Manuscript Releases,* vol. 1, 241)

"Those thus born again will go from our institution prepared to speak to others of Him who has done so much for them. Jesus says of them, 'Ye are my witnesses.' Isaiah 43:10. God grant them a renewal of life and health that they may go forth to impart to others the knowledge they have obtained, to tell their friends that they may keep well by eating temperately and drinking temperately, discarding TEA, COFFEE, DRUGS of all kinds, and ALCOHOL in all its forms. They go from the sanitarium as newborn souls, converted and enlightened, knowing that by being temperate in all things, and depending on Him who gave His life for them, they may work for God. . . .

"It is that such work as this may be done that we wish to establish a sanitarium. We ask you to give us a liberal donation. A great work can be accomplished for the Lord by a well conducted sanitarium. We have demonstrated this in America. To our sanitarium in America have come lawyers, doctors, senators, {87} and judges, to be guarded day and night against the cruel appetite for ALCOHOL, TOBACCO, and MORPHINE. Eternity alone can reveal the good that has been accomplished for them. They have gone forth to proclaim the glory of God and to do honor to His name."

1900—*Review and Herald,* November 6, 1900.

"No man or woman has any right to form habits which lessen the healthful action of one organ of mind or body. He who perverts his powers is defiling the temple of the Holy Spirit. The Lord will not work

a miracle to restore to soundness those who continue to use DRUGS which so degrade soul, mind, and body that sacred things are not appreciated. Those who give themselves up to the use of TOBACCO and LIQUOR do not appreciate their intellect. They do not realize the value of the faculties God has given them. They allow their powers to wither and decay."
(*Temperance,* 142)

1901—*The Southern Review,* January 1, 1901.

" 'Bless the LORD, O my soul: and all that is within me, bless his holy name,' (Psalm 103:1) because our guidebook is so very plain and definite. Others may not follow the plain 'It is written,' which Christ used on every occasion to meet the fallen foe, but let us follow the Saviour's example. The less we give expression to our human opinions, the purer and more marked with grace will be our conversation. The Lord calls for sanctified speech, because it is a savor of life unto life. He requires every human agent to take special care of his own soul-temple, allowing nothing that defileth to enter his lips, using no STIMULANTS or NARCOTICS, refusing to eat many kinds of food at meals, because thereby a cesspool is made of the stomach. God calls. Attention all! 'Watch ye, stand fast in the faith, quit ye like men, be strong.' 1 Corinthians 16:13. 'Be sober, be vigilant; because your adversary the devil, as a roaring lion, walketh about, seeking whom he may devour: whom resist steadfast in the faith, knowing that the same afflictions are accomplished in your brethren that are in the world. But the God of all grace, who hath called us unto his eternal glory by Jesus Christ, after that ye have suffered a while, make you perfect, stablish, strengthen, settle you. To him be glory and dominion for ever and ever.' 1 Peter 5:8–11."

1901—*Temperance,* 68.

"So powerful is the habit when once formed, that the use of TOBACCO becomes popular. An example of sin is set before youth, whose minds should be disabused of all thought that the use of the NARCOTIC is not harmful. They are not told of its injurious effects on the physical, mental, and moral powers."

1901—*The General Conference Bulletin,* April 12, 1901.

"Then, in after years, the light was given that we should have a sanitarium, a health institution, which was to be established right among us. This was the means God was to use in bringing His people to a right understanding in regard to health reform. It was also to be the means by which we were to gain access to those not of our faith. We were to have an institution where the sick could be relieved of suffering, and that without DRUG MEDICATION. God declared that He Himself would go before His people in this work."

(The Ellen G. White 1888 Materials, 1749; Notebook Leaflets from the Elmshaven Library, vol.1, 136; Counsels on Health, 531)

1901—*Counsels on Diet and Foods*, 106, 432.

"Hot drinks are not required, except as a MEDICINE. The stomach is greatly injured by a large quantity of hot food and hot drink. Thus the throat and digestive organs, and through them the other organs of the body, are enfeebled."

(Manuscript Releases, vol. 21, 286)

1901—*Manuscript Releases*, vol. 7, 12.

"I was much pleased with my visit to the Orphan's Home. I feel so thankful that the homeless can have so pleasant a home. I have never before seen gathered together so large a number of children, and all bright and cheerful. Their faces are healthy, their eyes clear, their nerves strong. To see them and hear them does me more good than a dose of MEDICINE. The superintendent seems to be well adapted to his position of trust, which he occupies with his wife."

1901—*The Use of Drugs in the Care of the Sick*, Ellen G. White Publications Manuscript, 41.

"There is one thing that has saved life—an INFUSION of BLOOD from one person to another; but this could be difficult and perhaps impossible for you to do. I merely suggest it."

1901—*Manuscript Releases*, vol. 8, 384.

"Concerning flesh meat we can all say, Let it alone. And all should bear a clear testimony against TEA and COFFEE, never using them. They are NARCOTICS, and are injurious to the brain and they clog the whole human machinery. It is also well to discard desserts. But we have not come to the time when I can say that the use of milk and eggs should be wholly discontinued. Milk and eggs should not be classed with flesh meat. In some ailments the use of eggs is necessary."

1901—*Manuscript Releases*, vol. 16, 147.

"Books relating to health and temperance could be placed in many homes. The circulation of these books is an important work; for they contain precious knowledge in regard to the treatment of disease—knowledge that would be a great blessing to those who cannot afford to pay for the physician's visits or for the DRUGS which, even if obtained, would be only an injury."

1901—*Manuscript Releases,* vol. 17, 91.

"While you were at Ann Arbor you gained wrong ideas in this respect. It would have been better if those sent from our schools to Ann Arbor had never had any connection with that institution. The education in DRUG MEDICATION and the false religious theories have brought forth a class of practitioners who need to unlearn much they have learned. They need to obtain an altogether different experience before they can say in word and in deed, We are medical missionaries. Till they obtain such an experience, the Great Physician does not acknowledge them as medical missionaries. They come onto the platform of action unprepared for the high and holy work which needs to be done at this time."

1901—*Manuscript Releases,* vol. 21, 285–286.

"Olives may be prepared in such a way that they will be superior to ANY DRUG in helping consumptives and those who have inflamed, irritated {286} stomachs. Olives might be eaten with good results at every meal. The advantage supposed to be gained by the eating of butter may be obtained by eating properly prepared olives. The oil in olives is a remedy for constipation and kidney diseases."

1901—*S.D.A. Bible Commentary,* vol. 3, 1151–1152.

"The words and works of the Lord harmonize. His words are gracious and His works bountiful. 'He causeth the grass to grow for the cattle, and HERB for the service of man.' Psalm 104:14. How liberal are the provisions He has made for us! How wonderfully He has displayed His munificence and power in our behalf! Should our gracious Benefactor treat us as we treat one another, where would we be? Shall we not strive earnestly to follow the golden rule, 'All things {1152} whatsoever ye would that men should do to you, do ye even so to them: for this is the law and the prophets.' Matthew 7:12."

1901—*Sermons and Talks,* vol. 2, 147.

"But the enemy will try to cast his dark shadow between our souls and God. He presents every possible inducement to lead us to be false to our Maker. He tries to gain control of the appetite, so that men and women shall make a god to the stomach. He knows that if they do this, their senses will become beclouded by overeating. He offers them STIMULANTS and NARCOTICS, hoping to lead them, in the use of these things, to forget God. Let us remember that these are the devices of the enemy to lead us to forget the advantages we may gain by every day eating the Bread of life."

1901—*Series B, No. 3a, Letters to Sanitarium Workers in Southern California*, 9 .

"The physicians present were interested in these words, and one, extending his arms and waving them back and forth, said, 'Is not this better than DRUGS? Aches and pains have left you, without the use of MEDICINE.' "

(*Series B, No. 3c, Letters From Ellen G. White To Sanitarium Workers in Southern California*, 9; *Manuscript Releases*, vol. 1, 247)

1902—*Counsels on Diet and Foods*, 402.

"Concerning flesh meat we can all say, Let it alone. And all should bear clear testimony against TEA and COFFEE, never using them. They are NARCOTICS, injurious alike to the brain and to the other organs of the body. The time has not yet come when I say that the use of milk and eggs should be wholly discontinued. Milk and eggs should not be classed with flesh meats. In some ailments the use of eggs is very beneficial."

(*Medical Ministry*, 274; *Testimony Studies on Diet and Foods*, 76;
FP—*Counsels on Diet and Foods*, 430; *Temperance*, 79; *Testimony Studies on Diet and Foods*, 150)

1902—*Pamphlet 144, The Place of Herbs in Rational Therapy*, 17–18.

"The Lord will be the Helper of every physician who will work together with Him {18} in the effort to restore suffering humanity to health, not with DRUGS, but with nature's remedies. Christ is the great physician, the wonderful Healer. He gives success to those who work in partnership with Him."

1902—*Manuscript Releases*, vol. 17, 353.

"This return to God's original design is infinitely better than DRUG MEDICATION. All this was opened before me last night. I was awake from nine o'clock. Finding that I could not sleep, I dressed and asked the Lord to help me write out the instruction He had given me.

Spirit of Prophecy References

"I was referred to Ezekiel's vision of the mighty river. 'These waters issued out toward the east country, and go down into the desert, and go into the sea: which being brought forth into the sea, the waters shall be healed. And it shall come to pass, that every thing that liveth, which moveth, whithersoever the rivers shall come, shall live: . . . And by the river upon the bank thereof, on this side and on that side, shall grow all trees for meat, whose leaf shall not fade, neither shall the fruit thereof be consumed: it shall bring forth new fruit according to his months, because their waters they issued out of the sanctuary: and the fruit thereof shall be for meat, and the leaf thereof for MEDICINE.' Ezekiel 47:8–9, 12. Let all physicians be wise to learn."

1902—*Review and Herald,* July 29, 1902.

"The Lord has appointed the youth to be His helping hand. If in every church they would consecrate themselves to Him, if they would practice self-denial in the home, relieving their careworn mother, the mother could find time to make neighborly visits; and when opportunity offered, they could themselves give assistance by doing little errands of mercy and love. Books and papers treating on the subject of health and temperance could be placed in many homes. The circulation of this literature is an important matter; for thus precious knowledge can be imparted in regard to the treatment of disease—knowledge that would be a great blessing to those who cannot afford to pay for a physician's visits, or for DRUGS which, even if obtained, are only an injury."

1902—*Spalding and Magan Collection,* 228–229.

"In a certain place, preparations were being made to clear the land for the erection of a sanitarium. Light was given that there is health in the FRAGRANCE of the PINE, the CEDAR, and the FIR. And there are several other kinds of trees that have MEDICINAL PROPERTIES {229} that are health promoting. Let not such trees be ruthlessly cut down. Better change the site of the building than cut down these evergreen trees. There are lessons for us in these trees. God's Word declares, 'The righteous shall flourish like the palm tree: he shall grow like a cedar in Lebanon.' Psalm 92:12. David says, 'I am like a green olive tree in the house of the Lord: I trust in the mercy of God for ever and ever.' Psalm 52:8."

(*The Paulson Collection of Ellen G. White Letters,* 17)

Spirit of Prophecy References

1902—*Selected Messages*, book 2, 301.

"The Lord has been giving me light in regard to many things. He has shown me that our sanitariums should be erected on as high an elevation as is necessary to secure the best results, and that they are to be surrounded by extensive tracts of land, beautified by flowers and ornamental trees.

In a certain place, preparations were being made to clear the land for the erection of a sanitarium. Light was given that there is health in the FRAGRANCE of the PINE, the CEDAR, and the FIR. And there are several other kinds of trees that have MEDICINAL PROPERTIES that are health promoting. Let not such trees be ruthlessly cut down. . . . Let them live." (MP—*Pamphlet 144, The Place of Herbs in Rational Therapy*, 25)

1902—*Manuscript Releases*, vol. 19, 48–51.

"Let the helpers in the institution fully understand that in their daily work they are gaining an education more valuable than anything which they could gain merely in a schoolroom. A practical training is worth far more than theoretical knowledge. The common words by which we know simple remedies are as useful as are the technical terms used by physicians for these same remedies. To request a nurse to prepare some CATNIP TEA, answers the purpose fully as well as would directions given to her in language understood only after long study.

"The Lord does not use words that are meaningless to the ordinary person. When Hezekiah was sick, the prophet Isaiah said, 'Let them take a LUMP of FIGS, and lay it for a plaster upon the boil, and he shall recover.' Isaiah 38:21. The Lord speaks in a language so plain that everyone can understand Him. In order to become a {49} competent nurse, it is not necessary to learn so many technical terms that are understood by comparatively few. To acquire a familiarity with these long words, students use much precious time that they could use otherwise to better profit. These difficult names are a device to cover up the nature of POISONOUS DRUGS. . . . {50}

This is why the physicians and nurses in our medical institutions should be those who abide in Christ; for through their connection with the Heavenly Physician their patients will be blessed. Those God-fearing workers will have no use for POISONOUS DRUGS. They will use the natural agencies that God has given for the restoration of the sick. Time and again I have told the workers in our sanitariums that from the light that God has given me I know that they need not lose one patient suffering from a fever, if they take the case in hand in time and use rational methods of treatment instead of DRUGS. . . . {51}

"When we are willing to have our own minds unsoldered, and resoldered by the melting influences of the Spirit of God, we shall understand with new enlightenment Christ's instruction to us as recorded in the fourteenth, fifteenth, sixteenth, and seventeenth chapters of John. Oh, how great are the possibilities that He has placed within our reach! He says, 'Whatsoever ye shall ask the Father in my name, he will give it you.' John 16:23. He promises to come to us as a Comforter to bless us. Why do we not believe these promises? That which we lack in faith we make up by the use of DRUGS. Let us give up the DRUGS, believing that Jesus does not desire us to be sick, and that if we live according to the principles of health reform, He will keep us well."

1902—*Temperance*, 35.

"Men on whom devolve grave responsibilities in safeguarding their fellow men from accident and harm, are often untrue to their trust. Because of indulgence in TOBACCO and LIQUOR, they do not keep the mind clear and composed as did Daniel in the courts of Babylon. They becloud the brain by using STIMULATING NARCOTICS, and temporarily lose their reasoning faculties. Many a shipwreck upon the high seas can be traced to LIQUOR DRINKING."
(*Manuscript Releases,* vol. 19, 280)

1902—*Testimonies*, vol. 7, 76–77.

"The things of nature are God's blessings, provided to give health to body, mind, and soul. They are given to the well to keep them well and to the sick to make them well. Connected with water treatment, they are more effective in restoring health than all the DRUG MEDICATION in the world. . . .

"Nature is God's physician. The pure air, the glad sunshine, the beautiful flowers and trees, the orchards and vineyards, and outdoor exercise amid these surroundings, {77} are health-giving—the elixir of life. Outdoor life is the only MEDICINE that many invalids need. Its influence is powerful to heal sickness caused by fashionable life, a life that weakens and destroys the physical, mental, and spiritual powers."
(*Counsels on Health,* 169–170; *Reflecting Christ,* 145)

1902—*Testimonies*, vol. 7, 85–86.

"Life in the open air is good for body and mind. It is God's MEDICINE for the restoration of health. Pure air, good water, sunshine, the

beautiful surroundings of nature—these are His means for restoring the sick to health in natural ways. To the sick it is worth more than silver or gold to lie in the sunshine or in the shade of the trees. . . . {86}
(*Counsels on Health*, 166; *Loma Linda Messages*, 477;
FP—*Medical Ministry*, 233; *My Life Today*, 135; *Manuscript Releases*, vol. 17, 349; *The Ellen G. White Biography*, 1900–1905, vol. 5, 360)

"In the effort made to restore the sick to health, use is to be made of the beautiful things of the Lord's creation. Seeing the flowers, plucking the ripe fruit, listening to the happy songs of the birds, has a peculiarly exhilarating effect on the nervous system. From outdoor life men, women, and children gain a desire to be pure and guileless. By the influence of the quickening, reviving, life-giving properties of nature's great MEDICINAL RESOURCES the functions of the body are strengthened, the intellect awakened, the imagination quickened, the spirits enlivened, and the mind prepared to appreciate the beauty of God's Word.
(*Counsels on Health*, 167)

1902—*Testimonies*, vol. 7, 134.

"Olives may be so prepared as to be eaten with good results at every meal. The advantages sought by the use of butter may be obtained by the eating of properly prepared olives. The oil in the olives relieves constipation; and for consumptives, and for those who have inflamed, irritated stomachs, it is better than ANY DRUG. As a food it is better than any oil coming secondhand from animals."
(*Counsels on Diet and Foods*, 349; *Counsels on Health*, 477; *The Health Food Ministry*, 34; *Testimony Studies on Diet and Foods*, 13, 124)

1902—*The Kress Collection*, 145.

"There are persons who would be more benefited by abstinence from food for a day or two every week than by any amount of MEDICINE or treatment or medical advice. To fast one day a week would be of incalculable benefit to them. It is foolish for one to keep on eating day after day, and yet wonder why he is in distress. Let such an one relieve himself from distress by changing his diet or by eating less. If he wills to do so, he can soon obtain relief."

1903—*Education*, 197.

"There is a physiological truth—truth that we need to consider—in the scripture, 'A merry [rejoicing] heart doeth good like a MEDICINE.' Proverbs 17:22."
(*My Life Today*, 151)

Spirit of Prophecy References

1903—*Loma Linda Messages*, 72.

"Workers—gospel medical missionaries—are needed now. We cannot afford to spend years in preparation. Soon doors now open to the truth will be forever closed. Carry the message now. Do not wait, allowing the enemy to take possession of fields now open before you. Let little companies go forth to do the work to which Christ appointed His disciples. Let them labor as evangelists, scattering our publications, talking of the truth to those they meet, praying for the sick, and, if need be, treating them, not with DRUGS, but with nature's remedies. Let the workers remember always that they are dependent on God. Let them not trust in human beings for wisdom, but in the One who declares, 'All power is given unto me in heaven and in earth.' Matthew 28:18. Thus we labored in the early history of the message."

1903—*Manuscript Releases*, vol. 13, 41.

"My brother, my sister, the Lord has greatly blessed you both. Your cheerful, happy temperament will be as a MEDICINE. Have faith in God. Move, step by step, onward and upward. And as you associate with the patients and minister to them by imparting God's Word of comfort and hope, may the words of truth be to them as a leaf from the tree of life. Lead them on to have faith in Jesus Christ. Thus many souls will decide to count the cost of their sinful indulgence of intemperate habits and sensual propensities—indulgence that, if continued, would prove the ruin of soul as well as of body."

1903—*The Use of Drugs in the Care of the Sick*, Ellen G. White Publications Manuscript, 30.

"Christ desires His people to be medical missionaries, able to do His will because they are acquainted with His principles of healing, and are prepared to use the remedies that He Himself has provided in the form of sunshine, pure air, and water. Thousands who go down to the grave might be healed if they would go to the LORD'S DISPENSARY rather than to the DRUGS that man provides."

1903—*Selected Messages*, book 2, 291.

"I have received much instruction regarding the location of sanitariums. They should be a few miles distant from the large cities, and land should be secured in connection with them. Fruit and vegetables should be cultivated, and the patients should be encouraged to take up outdoor work. Many who are suffering from pulmonary disease might be cured

if they would live in a climate where they could be out-of-doors most of the year. Many who have died of consumption might have lived if they had breathed more pure air. Fresh outdoor air is as healing as MEDI-CINE, and leaves no injurious aftereffects..
(*Spalding and Magan Collection, 257.*)

"It would have been better if, from the first, all DRUGS had been kept out of our sanitariums, and use had been made of such simple remedies as are found in pure water, pure air, sunlight, and some of the SIMPLE HERBS growing in the field. These would be just as efficacious as the DRUGS used under mysterious names, and concocted by human science. And they would leave no injurious effects in the system."
(*Pamphlet 144, The Place of Herbs in Rational Therapy, 15; Spalding and Magan Collection, 258; The Paulson Collection of Ellen G. White Letters, 40*)

"Thousands who are afflicted might recover their health if, instead of depending upon the DRUGSTORE for their life, they would discard all DRUGS and live simply, without using TEA, COFFEE, LIQUOR, or spices, which irritate the stomach and leave it weak, unable to digest even simple food without stimulation. The Lord is willing to let His light shine forth in clear, distinct rays to all who are weak and feeble."
(*Medical Ministry, 229; Temperance, 84; Testimony Studies on Diet and Foods, 85, 142, 149; The Paulson Collection of Ellen G. White Letters, 40; Spalding and Magan Collection, 258;
FP—Pamphlet 144, The Place of Herbs in Rational Therapy, 15*)

1903—*Selected Messages*, book 2, 298.

"I will tell you a little about my experience with CHARCOAL as a remedy. For some forms of indigestion, it is more efficacious than DRUGS. A little olive oil into which some of this powder has been stirred tends to cleanse and heal. I find it is excellent. PULVERIZED CHARCOAL from eucalyptus wood we have used freely in cases of inflammation."
(*The Paulson Collection of Ellen G. White Letters, 38;
FP—Pamphlet 144, The Place of Herbs in Rational Therapy, 24–25*)

1903—*Sons and Daughters of God*, 97.

"There are many who are not satisfied with the work that God has given them. They are not satisfied to serve Him pleasantly in the place that He has marked out for them, or to do uncomplainingly the work that He has placed in their hands. It is right for us to be dissatisfied with the way in which we perform duty, but we are not to be dissatisfied with the duty itself, because . . . in His providence God places before human beings service that will be as MEDICINE for their diseased minds. . . . Some He places where relaxed discipline and over-indulgence will not become their snare, where they are taught to appreciate the value of time, and to make the best and wisest use of it."

1903—*Temperance*, 24.

"Those who frequent the saloons that are open to all who are foolish enough to tamper with the deadly evil they contain, are following the path that leads to eternal death. They are selling themselves, body, soul, and spirit, to Satan. Under the influence of the drink they take, they are led to do things from which, if they had not tasted the MADDENING DRUG, they would have shrunk in horror. When they are under the influence of the LIQUID POISON, they are in Satan's control. He rules them, and they cooperate with him."
(*Manuscript Releases*, vol. 20, 83; LP—*Counsels for the Church*, 103)

1903—*The Paulson Collection of Ellen G. White Letters*, 17.

"Use nature's remedies—water, sunshine, and fresh air. Do not use DRUGS. DRUGS never heal; they only change the features of the disease."

1904—*The Ellen G. White Biography*, 1900–1905, vol. 5, 350.

"The situation of the sanitarium property is one of the most favorable that I have ever seen for this work. The spacious lawns, the noble trees, the beauty of the scenery all around, answer to the representations shown me of what our sanitariums ought to be. . . . The roads through the park are very well kept, and the scenery is lovely. I rode out every day, and I cannot find words to describe the beauty of what I saw. I enjoyed looking at the many DIFFERENT KINDS of TREES in the park, but most of all I enjoyed looking at the NOBLE PINE. There are MEDICINAL PROPERTIES in the FRAGRANCE of these trees."
(*Manuscript Releases*, vol. 8, 120)

1904—*Loma Linda Messages*, 40.

"The buildings secured for this work should be out of the cities, in rural districts, so that the sick may have the benefit of outdoor life. By the beauty of flower and field, their minds will be diverted from themselves, from their aches and pains, and they will be led to look from nature to the God of nature, who has provided so abundantly the beauties of the natural world. The convalescent can lie in the shade of the trees, and those who are stronger can, if they wish, work among the flowers, doing just a little at first, and increasing their efforts as they grow stronger. Working in the garden, gathering flowers and fruit, listening to the birds praising God, the patients will be wonderfully blessed. Angels of God will draw near to them. They will forget their sorrows. Melancholy and depression will leave them. The fresh air and sunshine, and the exercise taken, will bring them life and vitality. The wearied brain and nerves will find relief. Good treatment and wholesome diet will build them up and strengthen them. They will feel no need for HEALTH-DESTROYING DRUGS or for INTOXICATING DRINK."

(Series B, No. 3a, Letters to Sanitarium Workers in Southern California, 13–14; Series B, No. 3c, Letters From Ellen G. White To Sanitarium Workers in Southern California, 13–14; Manuscript Releases, vol. 1, 255–256)

1904—*Medical Ministry*, 40.

"The Lord would have our physicians cooperate with Him in their treatment of the sick, showing more faith and using fewer DRUGS. Let us rely upon God. Our faith is feeble, and our hearts remain unchanged. God would have a change take place. He says, 'A new heart also will I give you.' Ezekiel 36:26. When this promise is fulfilled to the people of God, the condition of things will be very different from what it now is."

(Manuscript Releases, vol. 19, 363–364)

1904—*Medical Ministry*, 296–297.

"Many act as if health and disease were things entirely independent of their conduct and entirely outside their control. They do not reason from cause to effect, and submit to {297} feebleness and disease as a necessity. Violent attacks of sickness they believe to be special dispensations of Providence, or the result of some overruling, mastering power; and they resort to DRUGS as a cure for the evil. But the DRUGS taken to cure the disease weaken the system.

If those who are sick would exercise their muscles daily, women as well as men, in outdoor work, using brain, bone, and muscle proportionately, weakness and languor would disappear. Health would take the place of disease, and strength the place of feebleness."

(Manuscript Releases, vol. 19, 230; The Paulson Collection of Ellen G. White Letters, 34)

1904—*Temperance*, 248.

"And as the sick are led to put forth physical effort, the wearied brain and nerves will find relief, and pure water and wholesome, palatable food will build them up and strengthen them. They will feel no need for HEALTH-DESTROYING DRUGS or INTOXICATING DRINK."

1904—*The Paulson Collection of Ellen G. White Letters*, 34.

"The Lord has greatly helped me healthwise. Difficulties that I have had for twenty-five years have been removed. I have used no MEDI-CINE, but for hours during the night season, when I was unable to sleep, I prayed for the healing power of God. I asked the Lord to restore my eyesight, to strengthen my heart, and to relieve the spinal difficulty. I have improved wonderfully. My health is better this winter than it has been for many years. The Great Physician has wrought in my behalf, and I praise His holy name."

1904—*Review and Herald,* August 11, 1904.

"Let the patients be taught that the breathing of pure air is necessary to health. Let there be facilities for the giving of rational treatment, so that there will be no necessity for the use of DRUGS. By wise methods the patients are to be led more and more to take outdoor exercise. Everyone who is recovering from sickness needs such exercise, in order that disease may be completely overcome, and health regained. When physical health has been restored, men and women are better able to exercise that faith in Christ which secures the health of the soul, bringing peace and rest and joy from the consciousness of sins forgiven."

1904—*Atlantic Union Gleaner,* September 7, 1904.

"During my stay here, I have had an opportunity to see a great deal of the surroundings of the sanitarium. The forty acres belonging to the institution are in the midst of the Middlesex Fells, a State reservation of three thousand five hundred acres. We have driven slowly through the park in every direction, looking with delight at the lake and the trees, and inhaling the HEALTH-GIVING FRAGRANCE of the PINES. It is delightful to ride through the forest. There are many beautiful drives, and much lovely scenery. I enjoy looking at the many DIFFERENT KINDS OF TREES in the forest, but most of all I enjoy looking at the noble pines. There are MEDICINAL PROPERTIES in the FRAGRANCE of these trees. 'Life, life,' my husband used to say when riding among the pines. 'Breathe deep, Ellen; fill your lungs with the fragrant, life-giving atmosphere.' "
(*Review and Herald,* September 29, 1904; *Series B, No. 13, The New England Sanitarium,* 5;
LP—*Manuscript Releases,* vol. 5, 178)

1905—*Counsels on Diet and Foods,* 281.

"Institutions for the care of the sick are to be established, where those who are suffering from disease may be placed under the care of God-fearing medical missionaries, and be treated without DRUGS. To these institutions there will come those who have brought disease upon themselves by improper habits of eating and drinking, and a simple, wholesome, palatable diet is to be provided. There is to be no starvation diet. Wholesome articles of food are to be combined in such a way as to make appetizing dishes."

1905—*Review and Herald,* March 23, 1905.

"Our sanitariums are one of the most successful means of reaching all classes of people. Christ is no longer in this world in person, to go through our cities and towns and villages healing the sick. He has commissioned us to carry forward the medical missionary work that He began; and in this work we are to do our very best. Institutions for the care of the sick are to be established, where men and women may be placed under the care of God-fearing medical missionaries, and be treated without DRUGS. To these institutions will come those who have brought disease on themselves by improper habits of eating and drinking. These are to be taught the principles of healthful living. They are to be taught the value of self-denial and self-restraint. They are to be provided with a simple, wholesome, palatable diet, and are to be cared for by wise physicians and nurses."
(*Counsels on Health,* 212)

1905—*The Ellen G. White Biography,* 1900–1905, vol. 5, 386.

"Suitable places must be provided to which we can bring the sick and suffering who know nothing of our people, and scarcely anything of Bible truth. Every effort possible is to be made to show the sick that disease may be cured by rational methods of treatment, without having recourse to DRUGS. Let the sick be separated from harmful surroundings and associations, and placed in our sanitariums, where they can receive treatment from Christian nurses and physicians."

1905—*Evangelism,* 534–535.

"The Lord has shown me that there should be sanitariums near many important cities. . . . Suitable places must be provided to which we can bring the sick and suffering away from the cities, who know nothing of our people, and {535} scarcely anything of Bible truth. Every effort possible is to be made to show the sick that disease may be cured by rational methods of treatment, without having recourse to INJURIOUS DRUGS. Let the sick be separated from harmful surroundings and associations, and placed in our sanitariums, where they can receive treatment from Christian nurses and physicians, and thus they become acquainted with the Word of God."

1905—*Loma Linda Messages*, 30.

"When the light came that we should have a sanitarium, the reason was plainly given. There were many who needed to be educated in regard to healthful living. A place must be provided to which the sick could be taken, where they could be taught how to live so as to preserve health. At the same time, light was given that the sick could be successfully treated without DRUGS. This was the lesson that was to be practiced and taught by physicians and nurses, and by all other medical missionary workers. DRUGS were to be discarded because when they are taken into the system, their aftereffects is very injurious. Many suffering from fevers have died as the results of the DRUGS administered. They might have been alive today had they been given water treatment by those competent to administer it."
(*Manuscript Releases*, vol. 7, 378;
FP—*The Ellen G. White Biography*, 1900–1905, vol. 5, 387)

1905—*Loma Linda Messages*, 78.

"An experienced Christian nurse in the sickroom will use the best remedies within her knowledge for restoring the sufferer to health. And she will pleasantly and successfully draw the one for whom she is working to Christ, the Healer of the soul as well as of the body. The lessons given, line upon line, here a little and there a little, will have their influence. The older nurses, whether they be men or women, should lose no opportunity of calling the attention of the sick to Christ. Those who care for the sick should be prepared to blend spiritual healing with physical healing. Let the nurses in our sanitariums show that in the solemn work of caring for the sick, they do not rely on DRUG MEDICATION, but on the power of Christ, and the use of the simple remedies that He has provided—the application of hot and cold water and simple, nourishing food, without INTOXICATING LIQUOR of any kind, with judicious exercise, and a putting away of all injurious practices. In treatment such as this there is health for the sick."

1905—*Temperance*, 59.

"The use of LIQUOR or TOBACCO destroys the sensitive nerves of the brain, and benumbs the sensibilities. Under their influence crimes are committed that would have been left undone had the mind been clear and free from the influence of STIMULANTS or NARCOTICS."

1905—*Temperance*, 66.

"Millions of dollars are spent for STIMULANTS and NARCOTICS. All this money rightfully belongs to God, and those who thus misappropriate His entrusted goods will someday be called to give an account of how they have used their Lord's goods."

1905—*Testimonies*, vol. 9, 168.

"Christ is no longer in this world in person, to go through our cities and towns and villages, healing the sick; but He has commissioned us to carry forward the medical missionary work that He began. In this work we are to do our very best. Institutions for the care of the sick are to be established, where men and women suffering from disease may be placed under the care of God-fearing physicians and nurses, and be treated without DRUGS."

(*Counsels on Health*, 393; *The General Conference Bulletin*, June 3, 1909.; *Series B, No. 8, Testimonies to the Church Regarding The Strengthening of Our Institutions and Training Centers*, 25; *Loma Linda Messages*, 64, 137, 384; *The Paulson Collection of Ellen G. White Letters*, 190)

1905—*The Indiana Reporter*, May 13, 1908.

"Why, asks one and another, is not prayer offered for the miraculous healing of the sick, instead of so many sanitariums being established? The Lord has opened this matter before me. Our sanitariums are established to educate in regard to right habits of living. This education every member of the remnant church needs. The light given me was that sanitariums should be established, and that in them DRUG MEDICATION should be discarded, and simple, rational methods of treatment should be employed for healing of disease. In these institutions people were to be taught how to dress, breathe, and eat properly—how to prevent sickness by proper habits of living."

(LP—*Testimony Studies on Diet and Foods*, 84, 111–112; *Counsels on Diet and Foods*, 303, 444)

1905—*The Ministry of Healing*, 126–127, 134.

"A practice that is laying the foundation of a vast amount of disease and of even more serious evils is the free use of POISONOUS DRUGS. When attacked by disease, many will not take the trouble to search out the cause of their illness. Their chief anxiety is to rid themselves of pain and inconvenience. So they resort to PATENT NOSTRUMS, of whose real properties they know little, or they apply to a physician for some remedy to counteract the result of their misdoing, but with no thought of making a change in their unhealth-

ful habits. If immediate benefit is not realized, another MEDICINE is tried, and then another. Thus the evil continues.
(*Counsels on Health,* 89)

"People need to be taught that DRUGS do not cure disease. It is true that they sometimes afford present relief, and the patient appears to recover as the result of their use; this is because nature has sufficient vital force to expel the POISON and to correct the conditions that caused the disease. Health is recovered in spite of the DRUG. But in most cases the DRUG only changes the form and location of the disease. Often the effect of the POISON seems to be overcome for a time, but the results remain in the system and work great harm at some later period.
(*Counsels on Health,* 89)

"By the use of POISONOUS DRUGS, many bring upon themselves lifelong illness, and many lives are lost that might be {127} saved by the use of natural methods of healing. The POISONS contained in many so-called remedies create habits and appetites that mean ruin to both soul and body. Many of the POPULAR NOSTRUMS called PATENT MEDI-CINES, and even some of the DRUGS dispensed by physicians, act a part in laying the foundation of the LIQUOR HABIT, the OPIUM HABIT, the MORPHINE HABIT, that are so terrible a curse to society.
(*Counsels on Health,* 89; *Maranatha,* 233)

"The only hope of better things is in the education of the people in right principles. Let physicians teach the people that restorative power is not in DRUGS, but in nature. Disease is an effort of nature to free the system from conditions that result from a violation of the laws of health. In case of sickness, the cause should be ascertained. Unhealthful conditions should be changed, wrong habits corrected. Then nature is to be assisted in her effort to expel impurities and to re-establish right conditions in the system.... {134}
(*Counsels on Health,* 90; *Temperance,* 85–86)

"While disordering his nerves and clouding his brain by the use of NARCOTIC POISONS, how can one be true to the trust reposed in him as a skillful physician? How impossible for him to discern quickly or to execute with precision!"
(*Temperance,* 70)

1905—*The Ministry of Healing,* 146.

"Thousands need and would gladly receive instruction concerning the simple methods of treating the sick—methods that are taking the place of the use of POISONOUS DRUGS. There is great need of instruction in regard to dietetic reform. Wrong habits of eating and the use of

unhealthful food are in no small degree responsible for the intemperance and crime and wretchedness that curse the world."
(Reflecting Christ, 246; A Call to Medical Evangelism and Health Education, 32–33; Review and Herald, May 9, 1912 and December 24, 1914; Evangelism, 525–526; Counsels on Health, 389)

1905—*The Ministry of Healing*, 235, 240.

"When the abuse of health is carried so far that sickness results, the sufferer can often do for himself what no one else can do for him. The first thing to be done is to ascertain the true character of the sickness and then go to work intelligently to remove the cause. If the harmonious working of the system has become unbalanced by overwork, overeating, or other irregularities, do not endeavor to adjust the difficulties by adding a burden of POISONOUS MEDICINES. . . . {240}

"Such exercise would in many cases be better for the health than MEDICINE. Physicians often advise their patients to take an ocean voyage, to go to some mineral spring, or to visit different places for change of climate, when in most cases if they would eat temperately, and take cheerful, healthful exercise, they would recover health and would save time and money."

1905—*The Ministry of Healing*, 241, 257.

"Courage, hope, faith, sympathy, love, promote health and prolong life. A contented mind, a cheerful spirit, is health to the body and strength to the soul. 'A merry [rejoicing] heart doeth good like a MEDICINE.' Proverbs 17:22. . . . {257}
(Mind, Character, and Personality, vol. 2, 647; Counsels on Health, 344)

"Good deeds are twice a blessing, benefiting both the giver and the receiver of the kindness. The consciousness of right-doing is one of the best MEDICINES for diseased bodies and minds. When the mind is free and happy from a sense of duty well done and the satisfaction of giving happiness to others, the cheering, uplifting influence brings new life to the whole being."

1905—*The Ministry of Healing*, 281.

" 'A merry [rejoicing] heart doeth good like a MEDICINE.' Proverbs 17:22. Gratitude, rejoicing, benevolence, trust in God's love and care—these are health's greatest safeguard. To the Israelites they were to be the very keynote of life."

Spirit of Prophecy References

1905—*The Ministry of Healing*, 295–296.

"In order to know what are the best foods, we must study God's original plan for man's diet. He who created man {296} and who understands his needs appointed Adam his food. 'Behold,' He said, 'I have given you every HERB yielding seed, . . . and every tree, in which is the fruit of a tree yielding seed; to you it shall be for food.' Genesis 1:29, A.R.V. Upon leaving Eden to gain his livelihood by tilling the earth under the curse of sin, man received permission to eat also 'the HERB of the field.' Genesis 3:18."

1905—*The Ministry of Healing*, 325, 333–335.

"Under the head of STIMULANTS and NARCOTICS is classed a great variety of articles that, altogether used as food or drink, irritate the stomach, poison the blood, and excite the nerves. Their use is a positive evil. Men seek the excitement of STIMULANTS, because, for the time, the results are agreeable. But there is always a reaction. The use of unnatural STIMULANTS always tends to excess, and it is an active agent in promoting physical degeneration and decay. . . . {333}

(*Counsels on Diet and Foods*, 339; *Temperance*, 73; *Testimony Studies on Diet and Foods*, 133)

"In the light of what the Scriptures, nature, and reason teach concerning the use of intoxicants, how can Christians engage in the raising of HOPS for BEER MAKING, or in the {334} manufacture of WINE or CIDER for the market? If they love their neighbor as themselves, how can they help to place in his way that which will be a snare to him? . . . {335}

(*Temperance*, 100)

"It must be kept before the people that the right balance of the mental and moral powers depends in a great degree on the right condition of the physical system. ALL NARCOTICS and UNNATURAL STIMULANTS that enfeeble and degrade the physical nature tend to lower the tone of the intellect and morals. Intemperance lies at the foundation of the moral depravity of the world. By the indulgence of perverted appetite, man loses his power to resist temptation."

(*Counsels on Diet and Foods*, 429; *A Call to Medical Evangelism and Health Education*, 38–39; *Testimony Studies on Diet and Foods*, 135, 146; *Pamphlet 136, Gospel Temperance Work*, 6;
FP—*Temperance*, 195)

1905—*The Ministry of Healing*, 339, 346.

"From so-called Christian lands the curse is carried to the regions of idolatry. The poor, ignorant savages are taught the use of LIQUOR.

Even among the heathen, men of intelligence recognize and protest against it as a DEADLY POISON; but in vain have they sought to protect their lands from its ravages. By civilized peoples, TOBACCO, LIQUOR, and OPIUM are forced upon the heathen nations. The ungoverned passions of the savage, stimulated by drink, drag him down to degradation before unknown, and it becomes an almost hopeless undertaking to send missionaries to these lands. . . . {346}
(Temperance, 230)

"The honor of God, the stability of the nation, the well-being of the community, of the home, and of the individual, demand that every possible effort be made in arousing the people to the evil of intemperance. Soon we shall see the result of this terrible evil as we do not see it now. Who will put forth a determined effort to stay the work of destruction? As yet the contest has hardly begun. Let an army be formed to stop the sale of the DRUGGED LIQUORS that are making men mad. Let the danger from the LIQUOR TRAFFIC be made plain and a public sentiment be created that shall demand its prohibition. Let the drink-maddened men be given an opportunity to escape from their thralldom. Let the voice of the nation demand of its lawmakers that a stop be put to this infamous traffic.

" 'If thou forbear to deliver them that are drawn unto death, and those that are ready to be slain; if thou sayest, Behold, we knew it not; doth not he that pondereth the heart consider it? and he that keepeth thy soul, doth not he know it?' And 'what wilt thou say when he shall punish thee?' Proverbs 24:11–12; Jeremiah 13:21."
(The Signs of the Times, November 27, 1907)

1905—*The Ministry of Healing*, 384.

"As children emerge from babyhood, great care should still be taken in educating their tastes and appetite. Often they are permitted to eat what they choose and when they choose, without reference to health. The pains and money so often lavished upon unwholesome dainties lead the young to think that the highest object in life, and that which yields the greatest amount of happiness, is to be able to indulge the appetite. The result of this training is gluttony, then comes sickness, which is usually followed by dosing with POISONOUS DRUGS."
(Counsels on Diet and Foods, 230; Testimony Studies on Diet and Foods, 53)

1905—*The Use of Drugs in the Care of the Sick*, Ellen G. White Publications Manuscript, 37.

"Institutions for the care of the sick are to be established, where those who are suffering from disease may be placed under the care of God-fearing physicians and nurses, and be treated without DRUGS."

1905—*Manuscript Releases*, vol. 18, 227–228.

"We felt a little disappointed, Brother Ballenger, that you could not accompany Brother Palmer to the meeting at Mountain View. But you were in the place where the Lord wanted you to be. Good is the Lord, and greatly to be {228} praised. If only souls will be converted from the error of their ways, and seek the Lord, and learn the science of preserving the health of the body and the soul! And where can they learn these much needed lessons as well as at our sanitariums, which the Lord has said should be established in many places. Lectures might be given to the multitudes, but while the words spoken would enlighten many minds, how can people understand fully without a practical knowledge? One patient, successfully treated, will have a testimony to bear of the virtue of the simple methods of treatment—the simple, healthful remedies that nature has provided without the use of ANY DRUGS."

1905—*Counsels on Health*, 469.

"When the light came that we should begin sanitarium work, the reasons were plainly given. There were many who needed to be educated in regard to healthful living. As the work developed, we were instructed that suitable places were to be provided, to which we could bring the sick and suffering who knew nothing of our people and scarcely anything of the Bible, and there teach them how to regain health by rational methods of treatment without having recourse to POISONOUS DRUGS, and at the same time surround them with uplifting spiritual influences. As a part of the treatment, lectures were to be given on right habits of eating and drinking and dressing. Instruction was to be given regarding the choice and preparation of food, showing that food may be prepared so as to be wholesome and nourishing, and at the same time appetizing and palatable."
(*Review and Herald*, December 16, 1909; *Series B, No. 13, The New England Sanitarium,* 9)

1906—*The Ellen G. White Biography*, 1905–1915, vol. 6, 36.

"I have had the situation opened to me, my brother, and the results for which a sanitarium should be conducted. The Boulder Sanitarium had, in the fear of God, taken the ground that our leading sanitariums have taken—

to discard meat, TEA, COFFEE, SPIRITUOUS LIQUOR, and the DRUG MEDI-CATIONS. Temperance principles had been taught in parlor lectures, and in other ways. Wholesome foods were served, and genuine health reform was taught. This institution should have had the right of way. But by the location of another sanitarium so nearby, the principles of which are in some respects quite different from those of the Boulder Sanitarium, difficulties will be presented which should not exist."
(*Manuscript Releases*, vol. 8, 451)

1906—*Sermons and Talks*, vol. 2, 279.

"Where are the watchmen? The Lord declares that unless the cities shall change their characteristics, the saloons will be replaced. In the calamity that befell San Francisco, the Lord designed to wipe out the saloons that have been the source of great evils; and yet the officiating guardians, the men who are placed in responsible positions, prove un-faithful to their trust by legalizing the sale of LIQUOR. POISONOUS DRUGS are mingled with the LIQUOR. Men form the habit of using these DRUGS, and the appetite for such things is very powerful."

1906—*Review and Herald*, October 25, 1906.

" 'As the days of Noe were, so shall also the coming of the Son of man be.' Matthew 24:37. The drunkenness and the crime that now prevail, have been foretold by the Saviour Himself. We are living in the closing days of this earth's history. It is a most solemn time. Everything betokens the soon return of our Lord. The very conditions we see in the great cities of our land; the mad acts of men whose minds have been inflamed by DRUGGED LIQUOR sold under sanction of human enact-ments; the dead and the dying whose destruction can be traced to the use of POISONOUS LIQUOR—all these evils are but a fulfillment of our Saviour's prophecy, whereby we may know that Jesus will soon appear in the clouds of heaven. . . .

"The people of San Francisco must answer at the judgment bar of God for the reopening of the LIQUOR SALOONS in that city. O that our cities might reform! In places where the judgments of Heaven have fallen, God is now proving those whose lives He has spared, as to whether they will continue to allow health and reason to be destroyed by the sale of madden-ing drink. Today, in many places, men are being tried in courts of justice, because under the influence of DRUGGED LIQUOR they have committed all manner of violence and sin. Satan looks on, highly gratified over the persis-tent determination of men to sell and use these POISONOUS DRINKS."

Spirit of Prophecy References

1906—*The Use of Drugs in the Care of the Sick*, Ellen G. White Publications Manuscript, 41.

Dr. Gibbs:

Dear Brother,—

"I have just received a letter from Brother Stephen Belden of Norfolk Island. He is afflicted with a cancer. Brother Alfred Nobbs, the elder of the Norfolk Island Church, has also been afflicted with what appeared to be a cancer. He went to Sydney, and his face and head were badly cut in removing the cancer. But he received little help, and he still continues to suffer greatly.

"Brother Stephen Belden has a cancer on his ear. I thought that if you would send him POWDERS at once, with directions for their use, Brother Belden and Brother Nobbs might both be benefited by their use.

"Will you kindly respond by sending the POWDERS as soon as you receive this letter?

"I am not well today, so cannot write much. I will send you this line, hoping that you will send the POWDERS." See Appendix A.

1906—*Manuscript Releases*, vol. 21, 139.

"And our sanitariums have been erected to supply a great necessity in healing the sick and suffering ones, and thus counterwork the work of Satan. And as in the miracles when Christ was in the world, we His followers are to discard DRUGS. We are to have faith, living faith, to read the Word, to inspire faith, to pray by the bedside of the sick, to talk faith. And Christ says, 'Go ye therefore, and teach all nations, baptizing them in the name of the Father, and of the Son, and of the Holy Ghost.' Matthew 28:19. Thus many are to be converted; the power of living faith is inspired in human hearts."

1907—*Temperance*, 262.

"In our public meetings in Australia we took special pains to present clearly the fundamental principles of temperance reform. Generally, when I spoke to the people on Sunday, my theme was health and temperance. During some of the camp meetings, daily instruction was given on this subject. In several places the interest aroused over our position on the use of STIMULANTS and NARCOTICS led the friends of temperance to attend our meetings and learn more of the various doctrines of our faith."

1907—*Review and Herald*, May 2, 1907.

"There are many who are not satisfied to serve God cheerfully in

the place that He has marked out for them, or to do uncomplainingly the work that He has placed in their hands. It is right for us to be dissatisfied with the way in which we perform duty, but we are not to be dissatisfied with the duty itself, because we would rather do something else. In His providence God places before human beings service that will be as MEDICINE to their diseased minds. Thus he seeks to lead them to put aside the selfish preference, which, if cherished, would disqualify them for the work He has for them. If they accept and perform this service, their minds will be cured. If they refuse it, they will be left at strife with themselves and with others."
(*Gospel Workers.* 270)

1907—*The Paulson Collection of Ellen G. White Letters*, 29–30.

"Our sanitariums are established as institutions where patients and helpers may serve God. We desire to encourage as many as possible to act their part individually in living healthfully. We desire to encourage the sick to discard the use of DRUGS, and to substitute the simple remedies {30} provided by God, as they are found in water, in pure air, in exercise, and in general hygiene."
(*Manuscript Releases,* vol. 1, 227 and vol. 11, 187; *Sermons and Talks,* vol. 2, 289)

1907—*The Paulson Collection of Ellen G. White Letters*, 295.

"Tuesday afternoon I met with the stockholders of the Paradise Valley Sanitarium. Their council meeting was held in the bowling alley. In coming out, we had to pass through the assembly room, where there was a large audience. Brother Burden asked me to stay, as they were speaking of the work of higher education that should be carried on in medical lines, but I thought it best not to do this. After I had climbed the long flight of stairs to my room on the third floor, which was the third time for that day. I found an article that I had written about a year ago, in reference to the establishment of a school of the highest order, in which the students would not be taught to use DRUGS in the treatment of the sick. With this I went downstairs again, and returned to the meeting."
(*Loma Linda Messages,* 309)

1907—*Review and Herald,* August 29, 1907.

"There needs to be a great reformation on the subject of temperance. The world is filled with self-indulgence of every kind. Because of the benumbing influence of STIMULANTS and NARCOTICS the minds of many are unable to discern between the sacred and the common. Their mental powers are weakened, and they cannot discern the deep spiritual things of the Word of God. . . .

(*Counsels on Health, 432; Pamphlet 136, Gospel Temperance Work, 4;*
FP—Temperance, 232)

"Shall there not be among us as a people a revival of the temperance work? Why are we not putting forth much more decided efforts to oppose the LIQUOR TRAFFIC, which is ruining the souls of men, and is causing violence and crime of every description? With the great light that God has entrusted to us, we should be in the forefront of every true reform. The use of DRUGGED LIQUORS is making men mad, and leading them to commit the most horrible crimes. Because of the wickedness that follows largely as the result of the use of LIQUOR, the judgments of God are falling upon our earth today. Have we not a solemn responsibility to put forth earnest efforts in opposition to this great evil?"

(*Counsels on Health, 432*)

1907—*The Signs of the Times*, November 20, 1907.

" 'As the days of Noe were, so shall also the coming of the Son of man be.' Matthew 24:37. The drunkenness and the crime that now prevail have been foretold by the Saviour. We are living in the closing days of this earth's history. It is a most solemn time. Everything betokens the soon return of Christ. The very conditions we see in the great cities of our land, the mad acts of men whose minds have been inflamed by DRUGGED LIQUOR sold under sanction of the rulers of the people, the dead and the dying whose destruction can be traced to the use of POISONOUS LIQUOR—all these evils are but a fulfillment of our Saviour's prophecy, whereby we may know that Jesus will soon appear in the clouds of heaven."

1907—*The Signs of the Times*, December 4, 1907.

"The people of San Francisco must answer at the judgment bar of God for the reopening of the LIQUOR saloons in that city. O that our cities might reform! In places where the judgments of heaven have fallen, God is now proving those whose lives He has spared as to whether they will continue to allow health and reason to be destroyed by the sale of maddening drink. Today, in many places, men are being tried in courts of justice, because, under the influence of DRUGGED LIQUOR, they have committed all manner of crime. Satan looks on, highly gratified over the persistent determination of men to sell and use these POISONOUS DRINKS."

Spirit of Prophecy References

1908— Selected Messages Book 2, 300

I am very sorry to learn that Sister C is not well. I cannot advise any remedy for her cough better than EUCALYPTUS and HONEY. Into a tumbler of HONEY put a few drops of the EUCALYPTUS, stir it up well, and take whenever the cough comes on. I have had considerable trouble with my throat, but whenever I use this I overcome the difficulty very quickly. I have to use it only a few times, and the cough is removed. If you will use this PRESCRIPTION, you may be your own physician. If the first trial does not effect a cure, try it again. The best time to take it is before retiring.

(*Manuscript Releases Volume Fourteen, 339;*
LP—*The Use of Drugs in the Care of the Sick,* Ellen G. White Publications Manuscript, 40)

1908—*Loma Linda Messages,* 110.

"The character of the buildings, the terraced hill, covered by graceful pepper trees, the profusion of flowers and shrubs, the tall shade trees, the orchards and fields—all combine to make this place meet fully the descriptions that I have given in the past of the place presented to me as the most perfect for sanitarium work. Everything at Loma Linda is fresh and wholesome and attractive. The patients could live out-of-doors a large part of the time. The land will serve as a school for the education of patients. By outdoor exercises and working in the soil, men and women will regain their health. Rational methods for the cure of disease will be used in a variety of ways. DRUGS will be discarded."

(*Series B, No. 3b, Letters From Ellen G. White To Sanitarium Workers in Southern California, 14; Series B, No. 3c, Letters From Ellen G. White To Sanitarium Workers in Southern California, 41; The Paulson Collection of Ellen G. White Letters, 194;*
LP—*Pamphlet 94, Testimonies and Experiences Connected with the Loma Linda Sanitarium and College of Medical Evangelists, 39*)

1908—*Loma Linda Messages,* 198.

"A wonderful responsibility rests upon those connected with the sanitariums established in His name for the treatment of the sick. This is to be done without the use of POISONOUS DRUGS. Those who become workers in the sanitariums are to believe the Words of Christ, 'Lo, I am with you alway, even unto the end of the world.' Matthew 28:20. Those who have the fear of God in the heart will cultivate a sweet disposition. Forbearance and courtesy will be manifested in the life. Duties will be faithfully discharged and in a way that will not leave a disagreeable impression on the minds of the sick or the well."

(*The Paulson Collection of Ellen G. White Letters, 227*)

Spirit of Prophecy References

1908—*Loma Linda Messages*, 388.

"We must have medical instructors who will teach the sciences of healing without the use of DRUGS. If physicians refuse to give their services unless they can be paid the highest wage, we shall not bribe them. We are to prepare a company of workers who will follow Christ's methods."

1908—*Loma Linda Messages*, 412, 440–441.

"Be very careful not to do anything that would restrict the work at Loma Linda. It is in the order of God that this property has been secured, and He has given instruction that a school should be connected with the sanitarium. A special work is to be done there in qualifying young men and young women to be efficient medical missionary workers. They are to be taught how to treat the sick without the use of DRUGS. Such an education requires an experience in practical work. The work at Loma Linda demands immediate consideration. Preparations must be made for the school to be opened as soon as possible. Our young men and young women are to find in Loma Linda a school where they can receive a medical missionary training, {441} and where they will not be brought under the influence of some who are seeking to undermine the truth. The students are to unite faithfully in the medical work, keeping their physical powers in the most perfect condition possible, and laboring under the instruction of the Great Medical Missionary. The healing of the sick, and the ministry of the Word, are to go hand in hand."

(FP—*The Paulson Collection of Ellen G. White Letters*, 218; *Pamphlet 95, Testimonies and Experiences Connected With The Loma Linda Sanitarium and College of Medical Evangelists*, 21; *Loma Linda Messages*, 182)

1908—*Loma Linda Messages*, 10.

"In the work of the school, maintain simplicity. No argument is so powerful as is success founded on simplicity. And you may have success in the education of students as medical missionaries without a medical school that can qualify physicians to compete with the physicians of the world. Let the students be given a practical education. And the less dependent you are upon worldly methods of education, the better it will be for the students. Special instruction should be given in the art of treating the sick without the use of POISONOUS DRUGS, and in harmony with the light God has given. Students should come forth from the school without having sacrificed the principles of health reform."

(LP—*The Medical Evangelist*, January 1, 1910; *Loma Linda Messages*, 316, 365, 413; *The Paulson Collection of Ellen G. White Letters*, 261; *Pamphlet 144, The*

Place of Herbs in Rational Therapy, 17; Pamphlet 61, Progress of Work at Loma Linda, 16)

1908—*Loma Linda Messages*, 441.

"In the work of the school, maintain simplicity. No argument is so powerful as is success founded upon simplicity. You may attain success in the education of students as medical missionaries without a medical school that can qualify physicians to compete with the physicians of the world. Let the students be given a practical education. The less dependent you are upon worldly methods of education, the better it will be for the students. Special instruction should be given in the art of treating the sick without the use of POISONOUS DRUGS and in harmony with the light that God has given. . . . In the treatment of the sick, POISONOUS DRUGS need not be used. . . Students should come forth from the school without having sacrificed the principles of health reform or their love for God and righteousness."

1908—*Medical Ministry*, 231.

"Those who desire to become missionaries are to hear instruction from competent physicians, who will teach them how to care for the sick without the use of DRUGS. Such lessons will be of the highest value to those who go out to labor in foreign countries. And the simple remedies used will save many lives."

(Health and Healing, 7; The Paulson Collection of Ellen G. White Letters, 35; Pamphlet 144, The Place of Herbs in Rational Therapy, 17)

1908—*Selected Messages*, book 2, 281.

"Nature's simple remedies will aid in recovery without leaving the deadly aftereffects so often felt by those who use POISONOUS DRUGS. They destroy the power of the patient to help himself. This power the patients are to be taught to exercise by learning to eat simple, healthful foods, by refusing to overload the stomach with a variety of foods at one meal. All these things should come into the education of the sick. Talks should be given showing how to preserve health, how to shun sickness, how to rest when rest is needed."

(Loma Linda Messages, 355; The Paulson Collection of Ellen G. White Letters, 37)

1908—*Selected Messages*, book 2, 288.

"The Lord has taught us that great efficacy for healing lies in a proper use of water. These treatments should be given skillfully. We have been instructed that in our treatment of the sick we should discard the use of DRUGS. There are SIMPLE HERBS that can be used for the

recovery of the sick, whose effect upon the system is very different from that of those DRUGS that poison the blood and endanger life."
(*Pamphlet 144, The Place of Herbs in Rational Therapy,* 15)

1908—*Selected Messages,* book 2, 295–296.

"There are many SIMPLE HERBS which, if our nurses would learn the value of, they could use in the place of DRUGS, and find very effective. Many times I have been applied to for advice as to what should be done in cases of sickness or accident, and I have mentioned some of these simple remedies, and they have proved helpful.
(*The Medical Evangelist,* January 1, 1910; *Loma Linda Messages,* 366; *The Paulson Collection of Ellen G. White Letters,* 35, 262; *Loma Linda Messages,* 366; FP—*Pamphlet 144, The Place of Herbs in Rational Therapy,* 16; *Loma Linda Messages,* 316)

"On one occasion a physician came to me in great distress. He had been called to attend a young woman who was dangerously ill. She had contracted fever while on the campground and was taken to our school building, near Melbourne, Australia. But she became so much worse that it was feared she could not live. The physician, Dr. Merritt Kellogg, came to me and said, 'Sister White, have you any light for me on this case? If relief cannot be given our sister, she can live but a few hours.' I replied, 'Send to a blacksmith's shop and get some PULVERIZED CHARCOAL; make a poultice of it, and lay it over her stomach and sides.' The doctor hastened away to follow out my instructions. Soon he returned, saying, 'Relief came in less than half an hour after the application of the poultices. She is now having the first natural sleep she has had for days.'
(*Pamphlet 144, The Place of Herbs in Rational Therapy,* 25–26; *The Paulson Collection of Ellen G. White Letters,* 36; *Loma Linda Messages,* 366)

"I have ordered the same treatment for others who were suffering great pain, and it has brought relief, and been the means of saving life. My mother had told me that snake bites and the sting of reptiles and poisonous insects could often be rendered harmless by the use of CHARCOAL POULTICES. When working on the land at Avondale, Australia, the workmen would often bruise their hands and limbs, and this in many cases resulted in such severe inflammation that the worker would have to leave his work for some time. One came to me one day in this condition, with his hand tied in a sling. He was much troubled over the circumstance; for his help was needed in clearing the land. I said to him, 'Go to the place where you have been burning the timber, and get me some CHARCOAL from the eucalyptus tree, pulverize it, and I will dress your hand.' This was {296} done, and the next morning he reported that the pain was gone. Soon he was ready to return to his work.

(*Pamphlet 144, The Place of Herbs in Rational Therapy,* 26–27; *The Paulson Collection of Ellen G. White Letters,* 36; *Loma Linda Messages,* 366)

"I write these things that you may know that the Lord has not left us without the use of simple remedies which, when used, will not leave the system in the weakened condition in which the use of DRUGS so often leaves it. We need well-trained nurses who can understand how to use the simple remedies that nature provides for restoration to health, and who can teach those who are ignorant of the laws of health how to use these simple but effective cures.

(*The Medical Evangelist,* January 1, 1910; *Loma Linda Messages,* 316–317, 366; *The Paulson Collection of Ellen G. White Letters,* 36, 262.)

"He who created men and women has an interest in those who suffer. He has directed in the establishment of our sanitariums and in the building up of schools close to our sanitariums, that they may become efficient mediums in training men and women for the work of ministering to suffering humanity. In the treatment of the sick, POISONOUS DRUGS need not be used. ALCOHOL or TOBACCO in any form must not be recommended, lest some soul be led to imbibe a taste for these evil things."

(*The Medical Evangelist,* January 1, 1910; *Loma Linda Messages,* 317, 367; *The Paulson Collection of Ellen G. White Letters,* 262)

1908—*Selected Messages,* book 2, 301–302.

"We need not go to China for our TEA, or to Java for our COFFEE. Some have said: 'Sister White uses TEA, she keeps it in her house;' and that she has placed it before them to drink. They have not told the truth because I do not use it, neither do I keep it in my house. Once when crossing the waters I was sick and could retain nothing on my stomach and I did take a little weak TEA as a MEDICINE, but I don't want any of you again to make the remark {302} that 'Sister White uses TEA.' If you will come to my house I will show you the bag that contains my HERB DRINK. I send to Michigan, across the mountains, and get the RED CLOVER TOP. In regard to COFFEE, I never could drink it, so those who reported that Sister White drinks COFFEE made a mistake."

1908—*Testimonies,* vol. 9, 175.

"The education that meets the world's standard is to be less and less valued by those who are seeking for efficiency in carrying the medical missionary work in connection with the work of the third angel's message. They are to be educated from the standpoint of conscience, and, as they conscientiously and faithfully follow right methods in their treatment of the sick, these methods will come to be recognized as preferable to the methods to which many have become accustomed, which demand the use of POISONOUS DRUGS."

(Pamphlet 61, Progress of Work at Loma Linda, 16; Loma Linda Messages, 413, 442)

1908—*Testimony Studies on Diet and Foods*, 86, 112.

"In our sanitariums, we advocate the use of simple remedies. We discourage the use of DRUGS, for they poison the current of the blood. In these institutions, sensible instruction should be given, how to eat, how to drink, how to dress, and how to live so that the health may be preserved."

(Counsels on Diet and Foods, 303; Selected Messages, book 2, 280; Sermons and Talks, vol. 1, 394; The Paulson Collection of Ellen G. White Letters, 35)

1908—*The General Conference Bulletin*, June 4, 1909.

"The education that meets the world's standard is to be less and less valued by those who are seeking for efficiency in carrying the medical missionary work in connection with the work of the third angel's message. They are to be educated from the standpoint of conscience, and, as they conscientiously and faithfully follow right methods in their treatment of the sick, these methods will come to be recognized as preferable to the method to which many have become accustomed, which demands the use of POISONOUS DRUGS."

(Testimonies, vol. 9, 175; The Medical Evangelist, January 1, 1910; Loma Linda Messages, 10, 316, 365; The Paulson Collection of Ellen G. White Letters, 261)

1908—*The Medical Evangelist*, April 1, 1910.

"It is not necessary that our medical missionaries follow the precise track marked out by the medical men of the world. They do not need to administer DRUGS to the sick. They do not need to follow DRUG MEDICATION in order to have influence in their work. The message was given me that if they would consecrate themselves to the Lord, if they would seek to obtain under men ordained of God a thorough knowledge of their work, the Lord would make them skillful. Connected with the divine Teacher, they will understand that their dependence is upon God and not upon the professedly wise men of the world."

(The Paulson Collection of Ellen G. White Letters, 307; Loma Linda Messages, 543–544)

Spirit of Prophecy References

1908—*The Paulson Collection of Ellen G. White Letters*, 36.

"This blending of our schools and sanitariums will prove an advantage in many ways. Through the instruction given by the sanitarium, students will learn how to avoid forming careless, intemperate habits of eating. Let the instruction be given in simple words. We have no need to use the many expressions used by worldly physicians, which are so difficult to understand that they must be interpreted by the physician. These long names are often used to conceal the character of the DRUGS being used to combat disease. We do not need these."

(Loma Linda Messages, 355)

1908—*The Paulson Collection of Ellen G. White Letters*, 40.

"If only our souls will be converted from the error of their ways, and seek the Lord, and learn the science of preserving the health of the body and the soul! And where can they learn these much-needed lessons as well as at our sanitariums, which the Lord has said should be established in many places? Lectures might be given to the multitudes, but while the words spoken would enlighten many minds, how can people understand fully without a practical knowledge? One patient, successfully treated, will have a testimony to bear of the virtue of the simple methods of treatment, the simple, healthful remedies that nature has provided, without the use of DRUGS."

1908—*The Paulson Collection of Ellen G. White Letters*, 261–262.

"There should be at our sanitariums intelligent men and {262} women, who can instruct in Christ's methods of ministry. Under the instruction of competent, consecrated teachers, the youth may become partakers of the divine nature, and learn how to escape the corruptions that are in the world through lust. I have been shown that we should have many more women who can deal especially with the diseases of women, many more lady nurses who will treat the sick in a simple way, and without the use of DRUGS."

(Pamphlet 61, Progress of Work at Loma Linda, 17; Loma Linda Messages, 10, 316, 366;
LP—Pamphlet 144, The Place of Herbs in Rational Therapy, 16; The Paulson Collection of Ellen G. White Letters, 1908)

1908—*The Paulson Collection of Ellen G. White Letters*, 266.

"The Lord calls for the best talents to be united at this center [Loma Linda] for the carrying on of the work as He has directed, not the talent that will demand the largest salary, but the talent that will place itself on the side of Christ to work in His lines.

"We must have medical instructors who will teach the science of healing without the use of DRUGS. If physicians refuse to give their services unless they can be paid the highest wage, we shall not bribe them. We are to prepare a company of workers who will follow Christ's methods."
(F & LP—*Medical Ministry*, 75;
LP—*Loma Linda's Work*, 10)

1908—*The Use of Drugs in the Care of the Sick*, Ellen G. White Publications Manuscript, 40.

"I have had considerable trouble with my throat, but whenever I use this [EUCALYPTUS and HONEY]. I overcome the difficulty very quickly. I have to use only a few times, and the cough is removed. If the first trial does not effect a cure, try it again. The best time to take it is before retiring."

1909—*Review and Herald*, January 14, 1909.

" 'Beside this, giving all diligence, add to your faith virtue; and to virtue knowledge; and to knowledge temperance.' 2 Peter 1:5–6. Here the importance of temperance is brought to our notice. Consider how the evil of intemperance is at work in our cities. Do we not know that the LIQUOR sold in the saloons of our land is DRUGGED with the most POISONOUS SUBSTANCES ? We read of one and another who has taken life while under the influence of LIQUOR—LIQUOR that has robbed them of their reason. We need to have a knowledge of these things that we may work intelligently to help others. The temperance cause needs to be revived as it has not yet been. We need to preach the gospel, that men and women may understand how to obey the Word of God. It is the Word of the living God that will bring men and women into right relation to Him; it will make impressions on heart and mind and character. Let every one of us be aroused to do the work that is waiting to be done—the work that Christ did when He was in the world. By beholding the works of Christ, humanity will take hold upon Divinity. There the appeal to souls is made, and He never turns one away. Whatever may be the position in life, whatever the past may have been, He will still receive."

1909—*Review and Herald*, January 21, 1909.

"We have a living Healer today. We need not depend upon DRUGS, but upon the Great Physician. If every sanitarium in our land were in living connection with God, the truth would go forth from our institutions as a lamp that burneth. They would carry mercy and light and compassion to the people, until men and women would realize that this is the religion of Christ, and that it reaches to suffering humanity."

1904–1909—*Ellen G. White Question and Answer File*, No. 34–B–2, Dr. S. P. S. Edwards letter to F. D. Nichol, November 24, 1957 as quoted in *Review and Herald*, July 7, 1983.

"This [QUININE in therapeutic doses with hydrotherapy to treat Malaria] (See Appendix B) is different from what I refer to in my testimonies. Like using ETHER or CHLOROFORM for surgery, you use one or two doses to kill the cause and do not continue to dose the patient day after day as is done in so many places. It is the repeated DRUGGING that I have condemned."

1909—*Medical Ministry*, 29.

"Christ declared that He came to recover men's lives. This work is to be done by Christ's followers, and it is to be done by the most simple means. Families are to be taught how to care for the sick. The hope of the gospel is to be revived in the hearts of men and women. We must seek to draw them to the Great Healer. In the work of healing let the physicians work intelligently, not with DRUGS, but by following rational methods. Then let them by the prayer of faith draw upon the power of God to stay the progress of disease. This will inspire in the suffering ones belief in Christ and the power of prayer, and it will give them confidence in our simple methods of treating disease. Such work will be a means of directing minds to the truth, and will be of great efficiency in the work of the gospel ministry."

1909—*Testimonies*, vol. 9, 168–169, 172.

"Let the Lord's work go forward. Let the medical missionary and the educational work go forward. I am sure {169} that this is our great lack—earnest, devoted, intelligent, capable workers. In every large city there should be a representation of true medical missionary work. Let many now ask: 'Lord, what wilt thou have me to do?' Acts 9:6. It is the Lord's purpose that His method of healing without DRUGS shall be brought into prominence in every large city through our medical institutions. God invests with holy dignity those who go forth farther and still farther, in every place to which it is possible to obtain entrance. Satan will make the work as difficult as possible, but Divine Power will attend all truehearted workers. Guided by our heavenly Father's hand, let us go forward, improving every opportunity to extend the work of God. . . . {172}

(*The General Conference Bulletin*, June 3, 1909; *Series B, No. 8, Testimonies to the Church Regarding The Strengthening of Our Institutions and Training Centers*, 26; *Loma Linda Messages*, 384–385; *Counsels on Health*, 393–394; LP—*Loma Linda Messages*, 53; *Medical Ministry*, 325)

"Workers—gospel medical missionaries—are needed now. We cannot afford to spend years in preparation. Soon doors now open to the truth will be forever closed. Carry the message now. Do not wait, allowing the enemy to take possession of the fields now open before you. Let little companies go forth to do the work to which Christ appointed his disciples. Let them labor as evangelists, scattering our publications, and talking of the truth to those they meet. Let them pray for the sick, ministering to their necessities, not with DRUGS, but with nature's remedies, and teaching them how to regain health and avoid disease."

(*The General Conference Bulletin*, June 3, 1909; *Series B, No. 8, Testimonies to the Church Regarding The Strengthening of Our Institutions and Training Centers*, 30–31; *Loma Linda Messages*, 58, 387; *Spalding and Magan Collection*, 320; *Christian Service*, 128; *Counsels on Health*, 397)

1909—*Testimonies*, vol. 9, 175–176.

"In the work of the school maintain simplicity. No argument is so powerful as is success founded on simplicity. You may attain success in the education of students as medical missionaries without a medical school that can qualify physicians to compete with the physicians of the world. Let the students be given a practical education. The less dependent you are upon worldly methods of education, the better it will be for the students. Special instruction should be given in the art of treating the sick without the use of POISONOUS DRUGS and in harmony with the light that God has given. In the treatment of the sick, POISONOUS DRUGS need not be used. Students should come forth from the school without having sacrificed the principles of health reform or their love for God and righteousness. . . . {176}

(*The General Conference Bulletin*, June 4, 1909; *Manuscript Releases*, vol. 11, 189)

"There should be at our sanitariums intelligent men and women who can instruct in Christ's methods of ministry. Under the instruction of competent, consecrated teachers the youth may become partakers of the divine nature and learn how to escape the corruption that is in the world through

lust. I have been instructed that we should have many more women who can deal especially with the diseases of women, many more lady nurses who will treat the sick in a simple way without the use of DRUGS."
(*The General Conference Bulletin,* June 4, 1909)

1909—*The General Conference Bulletin,* May 30, 1909.

"With all the precious light that has continually been given to us in the health publications, we cannot afford to live careless, heedless lives, eating and drinking as we please, and indulging in the use of STIMULANTS, NARCOTICS, and condiments. Let us take into consideration the fact that we have souls to save or to lose, and that it is of vital consequence how we relate ourselves to the question of temperance. It is of great importance that individually we act well our part, and have an intelligent understanding of what we should eat and drink, and how we should live to preserve health. All are being proved to see whether they will accept the principles of health reform or follow a course of self-indulgence."
(*Counsels on Diet and Foods,* 341; *Review and Herald,* February 10, 1910)

1909—*Manuscript Releases,* vol. 18, 234.

"In Oakland there has been for years a strong influence against the principles of health reform, which has counterworked the messages the Lord has given concerning the use of flesh meats and the use of DRUGS.

"When the Lord sent instruction regarding the principles of health reform and the dangers attending the use of flesh meats and the use of DRUGS, there were physicians standing in our sanitariums who chose to hold to their own ideas, to carry out their own plans for the table. They were opposed to the reforms that were called for, and indulgence of appetite was permitted in the rooms of the patients which was contrary to the principles for the maintenance of which our sanitariums were established."

1909—*The Kress Collection,* 165.

"The minds of the suffering ones must be led to grasp the hope of deliverance from special peril. Speak to them hopeful words, words of courage. There are those patronizing our sanitariums whom the Lord will heal if they will abstain from the use of LIQUOR and DRUGS, and will use simple and safe remedies to counteract disease brought on through perverted appetite. If they will act their part to break the spell of the enemy by firmly resisting temptation and will surrender themselves to the One who gave His life for sinful souls, they will become sons and daughters of God."

Spirit of Prophecy References

1909—*The Paulson Collection of Ellen G. White Letters*, 301.

"Intemperance and ungodliness are increasing everywhere. The work of temperance must begin in our own hearts. And the work of the physicians must begin in an understanding of the works and teachings of the great Physician. Christ left the courts of heaven that He might minister to the sick and suffering of earth. We must cooperate with the Chief of Physicians, walking in all humility of mind before Him. Then the Lord will bless our earnest efforts to relieve suffering humanity. It is not by the use of POISONOUS DRUGS that this will be done, but by the use of simple remedies. We should seek to correct false habits and practices, and teach the lessons of self-denial. The indulgence of appetite is the greatest evil with which we have to contend."

(*Loma Linda Messages*, 453; *The Medical Evangelist*, October 1, 1909; *Medical Ministry*, 85)

1909—*The Use of Drugs in the Care of the Sick*, Ellen G. White Publications Manuscript, 40.

"I have already told you the remedy I use when suffering from difficulties with my throat. I take a glass of BOILED HONEY, and into this I put a few drops of EUCALYPTUS OIL, stirring it in well. When the cough comes on, I take a teaspoonful of this mixture, and relief comes almost immediately. I have always used this with the best results. I ask you to use the same remedy when you are troubled with the cough. This PRESCRIPTION may seem so simple that you feel no confidence in it. but I have tried it for a number of years, and can highly recommend it."

(*Selected Messages*, Book 2, 301)

1909—*The Use of Drugs in the Care of the Sick*, Ellen G. White Publications Manuscript, 40.

"Take warm footbaths, into which have been put the LEAVES from the EUCALYPTUS TREE. There is great virtue in these leaves, and if you will try this, you will prove my words to be true. The OIL of the EUCALYPTUS is especially beneficial in cases of cough and pains in the chest and lungs. I want you to make a trial of this remedy which is so simple, and which costs you nothing."

1910—*Loma Linda Messages*, 554–555.

"In one of the most recent communications relative to this work, these

words occur, 'We are not to accept and follow the views of men who refuse to recognize God as their teacher, but who learn of men and are guided by man-made laws and restrictions. I was shown how that in a special sense we as a people {555} are to be guided by divine instruction. Those fitting themselves for medical missionary work should fear to place themselves under worldly doctors, to imbibe their sentiments and peculiar prejudices, and to learn to express their ideas and views. . . . It is not necessary that our medical missionaries follow the precise track marked out by medical men of the world. They do not need to administer DRUGS to the sick. They do not need to follow the DRUG MEDICATION in order to have influence in their work. The message was given me that if they would consecrate themselves to the Lord, if they would seek to obtain under men ordained of God, a thorough knowledge of their work, the Lord would make them skillful. . . . Some of our medical missionaries have supposed that a medical training according to the plans of worldly schools is essential to their success. To those who have thought that the only way to success is by being taught by worldly men and by pursuing a course that is sanctioned by worldly men, I would now say, put away such ideas. This is a mistake that should be corrected. It is a dangerous thing to catch the spirit of the world; the popularity which such a course invites, will bring into the work a spirit which the Word of God cannot sanction. It is a lack of faith in the power of God that leads our physicians to lean so much upon the arm of law, and to trust so much to the influence of worldly powers. The true medical missionary will be wise in the treatment of the sick, using the remedies that nature provides. And then he will look to Christ as the True Healer of diseases. The principles of health reform brought into the life of the patient, the use of nature's remedies and the cooperation of divine agencies in behalf of the suffering, will bring success."
(LP—*Review and Herald,* March 6, 1913)

1910—*Ellen G. White Question and Answer File,* No. 34–B–2, Dr. S. P. S. Edwards letter to F. D. Nichol, November 24, 1957 as quoted in *Review and Herald,* July 7, 1983.

"If QUININE will save a life, use QUININE." (See Appendix B).

1910—*The Paulson Collection of Ellen G. White Letters,* 43.

"Not a POISONOUS DRUG should be used. When you have a case that does not respond to the use of simple remedies, take it to the Lord in prayer. Talk to Him as the only One who can help. Quote simple scripture with tenderness and faith. As Christ's chosen physicians, speak His words, sometimes to convince of sin, but always to inspire hope. When laboring for the patients, consider that their sensibilities must be awakened to the fact that Christ came to our world to save perishing souls."

1911—*Manuscript Releases,* vol. 1, 248.

"The object that we have in view is not to get money, particularly, it is to get souls, to take those who are suffering with disease, and place them in the best position possible for the recovery of health. We have no confidence in DRUG MEDICATION. God wants us to be out where we can have the advantages of nature in every respect, in the air and in the scenery."
(*Manuscript Releases,* vol. 10, 250)

1911—*Loma Linda Messages,* 581.

"Our people should become intelligent in the treatment of sickness without the aid of POISONOUS DRUGS. Many should seek to obtain the education that will enable them to combat disease in its varied forms by the most simple methods. Thousands have been restored to health by simple methods of treatment. Let diligent study be united with faithful ministry. Let prayers of faith be offered by the bedside of the sick. Let the sick be encouraged to claim the promises of God for themselves. 'Faith is the substance of things hoped for, the evidence of things not seen.' Hebrews 11:1. Christ Jesus, the Saviour of men, is to be brought into our labors and councils more and more."

1911—*Lake Union Herald,* September 13, 1911.

"Our people should become intelligent in the treatment of sickness without the aid of POISONOUS DRUGS. Many should seek to obtain the education that will enable them to combat disease in its varied forms by the most simple methods. Thousands have gone down to the grave because of the use of POISONOUS DRUGS, who might have been restored to health by the simple methods of treatment. Water treatments, wisely and skillfully given, may be the means of saving many lives. Let diligent study be united with faithful ministry. Let prayers of faith be offered by the bedside of the sick. Let the sick be encouraged to claim the promises of God for themselves. 'Faith is the substance of things hoped for, the evidence of things not seen.' Hebrews 11:1. Christ Jesus, the Saviour of men, is to be brought into our labors and councils more and more."
(*Pamphlet 9, An Appeal in Behalf of Our New Medical College,* 2.
FP—*Medical Ministry,* 57, 227)

Spirit of Prophecy References

1912—*Sermons and Talks*, vol. 2, 333.

"Looking upon the church members who are using the NARCOTIC TOBACCO, God says to them, 'Be ye clean, that bear the vessels of the LORD.' Isaiah 52:11."

1912—*Review and Herald*, April 25, 1912.

"The Saviour sought the people where they were, and placed before them the great truths of His kingdom. As He went from place to place, He blessed and comforted the suffering, and healed the sick. This is our work. Small companies are to go forth to do the work to which Christ appointed His disciples. While laboring as evangelists, they can visit the sick, praying with them, and if need be, treating them, not with MEDICINES, but with the remedies provided in nature."

1912—Manuscript Releases Volume Three, 323

We are sorry to hear that —— has met with so serious an accident. I have often found the application of EUCALYPTUS LEAVES to a wounded part to be good in allaying inflammation and drawing out the poison.

1913—*Counsels to Parents, Teachers, and Students*, 125–126.

"Children are to be trained to understand that every organ of the body and every faculty of the mind is the gift of a good and wise God, and that each is to be used to His {126} glory. Right habits in eating and drinking and dressing must be insisted upon. Wrong habits render the youth less susceptible to Bible instruction. The children are to be guarded against the indulgence of appetite, and especially against the use of STIMULANTS and NARCOTICS. The tables of Christian parents should not be loaded down with food containing condiments and spices."
(*Temperance*, 185;
LP–*Child Guidance*, 364)

1913—*Counsels to Parents, Teachers, and Students*, 469.

"I have been instructed that little companies who have received a suitable training in evangelical and medical missionary lines should go forth to do the work to which Christ appointed His disciples. Let them labor as evangelists, scattering our publications, talking of the truth to those they meet, praying for the sick, and, if need be, treating them, not with DRUGS, but with nature's remedies, ever realizing their dependence on God. As they unite in the work of teaching and healing they will reap a rich harvest of souls."
(*Notebook Leaflets from the Elmshaven Library*, vol.1, 140–141)

1913—*Loma Linda Messages*, 621—William. C. White to Ellen G. White.

"In New Castle, you remember, we were down there one time when Brother Starr and others were holding meetings. One Friday afternoon you and I were walking out by the creek, and you said that there was a reformation that we must stand for, in medical practice that was just as important as the discarding of DRUGS, and that was, the matter of very high charges for medical service."

1914—*Review and Herald*, December 17, 1914.

"Christ sought the people where they were, and placed before them the great truths in regard to His kingdom. As He went from place to place, He blessed and comforted the suffering and healed the sick. This is our work. Small companies are to go forth to do the work to which Christ appointed His disciples. While laboring as evangelists, they can visit the sick, praying with them, and if need be, treating them, not with MEDICINES, but with the remedies provided in nature."
(*Counsels on Health*, 501)

1915—*Gospel Workers*, 163–164.

"Rash, overbearing expressions do not harmonize with the sacred work that Christ has given His ministers to do. When the daily experience is one of looking unto Jesus and learning of Him, you will reveal a wholesome, harmonious character. Soften your representations, and let not condemnatory words be spoken. Learn of the great Teacher. Words of kindness and sympathy will do good as a MEDICINE, and will heal souls that are in despair. The knowledge of the Word of God brought into the practical life will have a healing, soothing power. Harshness of speech {164} will never bring blessing to yourself or to any other soul."

1915—*The Signs of the Times*, August 10, 1915.

"TOBACCO weakens the brain, and paralyzes its fine sensibilities. Its use excites a thirst for drink, and in very many cases, lays the foundation for the LIQUOR HABIT. Its use is an inconvenient, expensive, unclean habit. The teachings of Christ, pointing to purity, self-denial, and temperance, all rebuke this defiling practice. When we think of the long fast that Jesus endured in the wilderness of temptation in order to break the power of appetite over man, we marvel that those who profess to be His followers can indulge in this habit. Is it for the glory of God for men to enfeeble the physical powers, confuse the brain, and yield the will to this NARCOTIC POISON? What right have they to mar the image of God?"

19??—*Loma Linda Messages*, 238.

"In our public meetings in Australia, we took special pains to present clearly the fundamental principles of temperance reform. Generally, when I spoke to the people on Sunday, my theme was health and temperance. During some of the camp meetings, daily instruction was given on this subject. In several places, the interest aroused over our position on the use of STIMULANTS and NARCOTICS, led the friends of temperance to attend our meetings and learn more of the various doctrines of our faith."

Date?—*The Use of Drugs, A Statement Prepared Under the Direction of the General Conference Committee*, 16–17—D. E. Robinson, an E. G. White Secretary.

"You ask for definite and concise information regarding what Sister White wrote about VACCINATION and SERUM.

"This question can be answered very briefly for so far as we have any record, she did not refer to them in any of her writings.

"You will be interested to know, however, that at a time when there was an epidemic of smallpox in the vicinity, she herself was vaccinated and urged her helpers, those connected with her, to be vaccinated. In taking this step Sister White recognized the fact that it has been proven that VACCINATION either renders one immune from smallpox or greatly lightens its effects if one does come down with it. She also recognized the danger of their exposing others if they failed to take this precaution. . . .

"An uncle of mine, Elder D. A. Robinson, who labored as a missionary in India, was conscientiously opposed to VACCINATION and refused to take it. He died an awful death with smallpox, and before he died he stated that he had made a mistake which was costing him his life. The rest of the family were vaccinated, and suffered no ill effects from smallpox."

(FP—*Selected Messages*, book 2, 303 footnote)

Spirit of Prophecy References

Appendix A

The following are comments by the compilers of the cited Ellen G. White references, and appeared as footnotes or as introductory material in the publication.

Page 82. To understand the context in which Ellen White commented on the use of medicines and drugs, see the pamphlet entitled, "The Use of Drugs," issued by the General Conference: also three articles on Ellen White and modern medicine, in the *Adventist Review*, June 30, July 7, and July 14, 1983.

Page 101. The reader should keep in mind that the medications referred to here were poisonous substances that when taken into the body left lasting, harmful effects and were quite unrelated to many of the medications employed now in the treatment of the sick.

Page 107. Mrs. White is here referring to the 'General Practitioner' of 1897 in the backwoods of Australia, from where she penned these words. The reader must keep in mind that until the second decade of the twentieth century, physician training was largely unregulated and was often meager. In many instances it was on an apprentice basis, supplemented at best by a short period of training in a more or less orthodox medical school. The medical profession was without well-established standards. The mainstay in the medications of the ordinary doctor was poisonous drugs, often prescribed in large doses. The following facts show clearly that Mrs. White's statement should not be used to depreciate the labors of the carefully trained conscientious physician:

    1. Her many statements relative to the high calling and weighty responsibilities of the physician;

    2. Her practice of consulting qualified physicians as attested by the published record and by those who were members of her family;

    3. Her counsel to an associate worker who was ill, to 'let the physicians' 'do those things' for her 'that must be done' (see *Selected Messages*, book 2, 251), and urging her to eat, 'because your earthly physician would have you eat' (Ibid., 253);

4. Her many counsels addressed to practicing physicians presented in *The Ministry of Healing, Counsels on Health*, and *Medical Ministry*;

5. The guidance from her pen in the establishment of a Seventh-day Adventist Medical College at Loma Linda, designed to provide 'a medical education that will enable' its graduates 'to pass the examinations required by law of all those who practice as regularly qualified physicians.'—Ellen G. White Manuscript 7, 1910 (published in *Pacific Union Recorder*, Feburary 3, 1910). (See *The Story of Our Health Message* (1955), 386.)

Page 118. It is an interesting fact that as a result of twentieth century medical research, physicians have largely discarded most of the medications in common use at the time referred to in this statement.

Page 118. It is to be observed that a large proportion of the prescriptions written by the physicians of today call for ingredients taken from the vegetable kingdom, most of which are nonpoisonous.

Page 118. The Freemasons are a secret society based on the principles of brotherliness, charity, and mutual aid. Apparently Ellen White saw a parallel between the spirit of the close-knit medical fraternity and that of the Freemasons.

Page 151. The value of this communication lies, not in the powder Dr. Gibbs might suggest which might bring relief in the cancer case, but in the fact that Mrs. White was eager to have use made of a powder she hoped might be a remedy.

Appendix A

Appendix B

Ellen G. White Question and Answer File, No. 34–B–2, Dr. S. P. S. Edwards letter to F. D. Nichol, November 24, 1957 as quoted in *Review and Herald*, July 7, 1983.

Elder F. D. Nichol
Editor of Review and Herald,
Washington, D.C.

Dear Brother:

I have just read the second article on the "Use of Drugs" as printed in the *Review* of November 21. As I read the statements in regard to the use of QUININE, the following story came to me, and I decided to send it to you as it might help someone.

From 1904 to 1909 I was Medical Superintendent. of the Tri-City Sanitarium at Moline, Illinois. Being located on the Mississippi River there were many cases of malaria. Because of Sister White's statement about the use of QUININE, I refused to use it myself or give it to patients. With physiotherapy we were able to control the symptoms of malaria, but could not cure it. Most of those living along the river took QUININE daily as they ate their breakfast. The QUININE, in the doses usually taken, did no more for the patients than our physiotherapy treatments did. It was palliative only. Several of our doctors discussed the matter and decided that if one or two large doses of QUININE were given so as to saturate the blood, we could destroy the parasites in the blood and thus cure the disease. I tried it on a severe case of Tirtian Malaria. The patient was given 20 grains of QUININE the night before his chill was due, and he was put to bed with cold to his head. The next morning, two hours before time for the chill, he was given the same dose and immediately put in a continuous hot bath, and kept there till two hours after time for the chill. He did not have a chill then nor after, and his blood showed no signs of parasites. The hot bath caused him to sweat the QUININE out of his system so he had no bad after symptoms from the QUININE. This was repeated in many cases and never a failure.

Appendix B

Sister White visited the Sanitarium some time after this experience, and in course of our visits, I told her of my use of QUININE. She said in substance: "This is different from what I refer to in my Testimonies. Like using ETHER or CHLOROFORM for surgery, you use one or two doses to kill the cause and do not continue to dose the patient day after day as is done in so many places. It is the repeated drugging that I have condemned."

In 1910 I was at the St. Helena Sanitarium. One day W. C. White came to my room, and handing me a letter said that Mother had received this letter and wished me to answer it, telling the story I told her at Moline about the use of QUININE. The letter was from Elder J. E. Fulton in the South Sea Islands. He stated that workers and members were dying of malaria. Because of the statements in the Testimonies, they were not taking QUININE, and the hydrotherapy treatments were only palliative. "Tell us what to do." In my answer I told the Moline story and gave advice as to after treatment. I took the letter to Sister White and, after reading my answer, she took her pen and wrote a P.S. across the bottom of my letter as follows: "If QUININE will save a life, use QUININE. Ellen G. White." The letter was sent at once.

Fifteen years after that, I met Elder Fulton at a camp meeting in California, and he handed me a much worn envelope. On opening it, I found my letter of 1910 with the P.S. by Sister White. Said Elder Fulton, "That letter has been my constant companion and has saved many lives." Elder Eric Hare and wife can verify the receipt of the letter and its contents as they were there.

So far as I know this has never been told publicly. I have told it to those who have sought advice about drugs and their use, mostly doctors. I think that the copy without the P.S. is in the files at the vault. I am glad to see the statement about the use of DRUGS. Excuse mistakes as an old man is sure to make them.

God bless you in your ministry ,

(Signed) S. P. S. Edwards, M.D.

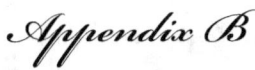

Appendix B

Appendix C

A Letter by Dr. Paulson on the Use of Drugs

Hinsdale, Illinois
July 9, 1914

Dr. Thyna H. Jasselyn
Madison, Ind.

Dear Doctor:

A few weeks ago Brother L. A. Hansen, of the Medical Missionary Department, forwarded to me the following questions which you had raised:

"I cannot understand what Mrs. White means when she says that DRUGS are not necessary in the treatment of disease unless it is just what she says, but I am told by another Adventist doctor on our staff that I misunderstood her attitude.

"Though I too think that we should not use DRUGS needlessly, I should not wish to disregard the value of ANTITOXIN in diphtheria, QUININE in malaria, etc.

"Other Adventist physicians use such remedies, and do not feel that they are in the wrong. I do not see how they reconcile their position with such statements as I enclose."

Brother Hansen suggested my writing something on this question. It is with some hesitancy that I do so because I feel that on a question of such vital importance if any man speak let him speak as the oracles of God (see 1 Peter 4:11), and unless God by His grace shall enable me to do that, I feel silence would be golden on my part.

We are naturally inclined to interpret the Testimonies in the light of our own practice instead of humbly acknowledging that we have come short of the glory of God. It is God's plan that the prophets should hew us up to the divine standard (see Hosea 6:5), while the tendency of our natural inclinations is to hew the prophets down to the level of our practice. On this question of DRUG therapy I am quite convinced that the reformers need to be reformed, that in brokenness of heart, like Daniel of old, we need to confess not only the sins of our medical brethren, but our own individual sins as well.

Some twenty-odd years ago a group of us medical students left the Battle Creek Sanitarium, and went to Ann Arbor to begin our medical course. Some of us made a most careful and prayerful study from the Bible and the Testimonies of fundamental medical missionary principles including, of course, therapeutics. We soon became convinced that there were some remedies that God had promised to especially bless, and that there were others to which He could not in a similar manner add His blessing.

Dr. Osler, now of Oxford, England, but then of Johns Hopkins, had just issued his first edition of his famous textbook on the practice of medicine. It was the most radical departure from the old therapeutic program that had ever appeared, and he speedily and justly earned the title of a therapeutic annihilist as far as DRUGS were concerned. It was evident to any careful observer that Dr. Osler placed little or no reliance in DRUG THERAPY. This naturally made it easier for some of us to take the various statements in the Testimonies more nearly at their par value.

Some of our number naturally undertook to harmonize these statements with their particular modified beliefs on the question. This led Brother Caro, my roommate, to write to Sister White some questions very similar to the ones you have raised. I am enclosing you a copy of her entire reply as far as it had any bearing whatsoever on this subject. Summed up in a nutshell, there is no repudiation of the former statements made; rather, the enunciation of this self-evident principle that the SIMPLER REMEDIES are less harmful in proportion to their simplicity, and that there are "HERBS and ROOTS" that every family may use for themselves as opposed to "DANGEROUS CONCOCTIONS." In a later unpublished testimony, written August 26, 1895, I quote the following:

"Many physicians in our world are of no benefit to the human family. The DRUG SCIENCE has been exalted, but if every bottle that comes from every such institution were done away with, there would be fewer invalids in the world today. DRUG MEDICATION should never have been introduced into our institutions. There was no need of this being so, and for this reason the Lord would have us establish an institution where He can come in and where His grace and power can be revealed. 'I am the resurrection, and the life,' He declares. John 11:25.

"The true method of healing the sick is to tell them of the HERBS that grow for the benefit of man. Scientists have attached large names to these simplest preparations, but true education will lead us to teach the sick that they need not call in a doctor any more than they would call in

Appendix C

a lawyer. They can themselves administer the SIMPLER HERBS if necessary. To educate the human family that the doctor alone knows all the ills of infants and persons of every age is false teaching, and the sooner we as a people stand on the principles of health reform, the greater will be the blessing that will come to those who would do true medical work. There is a work to be done in treating the sick with water, and teaching them to make the most of sunshine and physical exercise. Thus in simple language we may teach the people how to preserve health, how to avoid sickness. This is the work our sanitariums are called upon to do. This is true science." *Spalding and Magan's Unpublished Manuscript Testimonies*, 139–140. (All emphasis supplied unless otherwise noted.)

Here is a clean-cut statement that DRUG MEDICATION should never have been introduced into our institutions. At the same time, the point is emphasized that there are HERBS that grow for the benefit of man. The administering of these "SIMPLE HERBS if necessary" is put alongside the standing "on the principles of health reform," "treating the sick with water," and "sunshine and physical exercise."

It is evident even after all this instruction has been imparted to us on the subject of DRUG MEDICATION that there is still as always is the case, a twilight zone where the human agent must use his own sanctified judgment in making the full application. The Lord never deals with us in arbitrary terms. He still leaves plenty of necessity of seeking Him for individual light. It is very evident that, humanly speaking, it would be much more desirable if the Testimonies should have specifically pointed out SENNA, for instance, as a SIMPLE HERB that might properly be used, while on the other hand NUX VOMICA, as the Testimonies have already stated, is a DRUG that never should be used.

However, as I have stated above, much of the Lord's instruction is in general principles sufficiently plain that those who earnestly desire to do His will at any cost may, by the aid of the Holy Spirit, learn to apply it, while those who want to follow their own inclinations will have abundant excuse for doing so.

Instead of finishing at the University of Michigan, I graduated at Bellevue Medical College, New York City. The learned professor of medicine enthusiastically recommended ALCOHOL as the important remedy in various infectious diseases. Knowing that the Bible had declared it to be a deceiver, and that the Testimonies had unqualifiedly condemned it, all this false instruction did not influence me a hair's breadth. Naturally it is gratifying to me to have lived long enough to find no intelligent,

Appendix C

up-to-date physician today who believes ALCOHOL is anything but a detriment in the sickroom.

When we became physicians in the Battle Creek Sanitarium, some of us earnestly insisted that such DRUGS as STRYCHNINE, CALOMEL, and others that had been specifically pointed out as always injurious to the human system should be repudiated by the institution. I am glad to say that Dr. Kellogg, took the same position, and said that he never had any faith in them, that they had been dragged into the institution by some of the practitioners who had been taught in medical schools that they were valuable remedies.

Naturally the argument that MORPHINE was justifiable and essential to subdue the pain after an operation as was CHLOROFORM during an operation seemed unanswerable, and perhaps is yet in some instances unanswerable. However, I remember more than one case where even at the midnight hour some of us gathered in some quiet room and unitedly presented some poor sufferer's case to God in prayer, and were gratified to find ere we had finished our prayer the patient had dropped off into a sweet refreshing sleep from which he awoke entirely free from pain.

Mind you, none of us took the position that MORPHINE should never be used. We simply insisted, knowing its dangerous character, having abundant opportunity to see the poor DRUG SLAVES as they were drifting in there to be cured of its awful tyranny, that MORPHINE should not be injected into a patient until God's remedies, prayerfully applied, had had a fair opportunity to demonstrate what was God's will in that particular case.

Naturally QUININE was considered just as indispensable in malaria as MORPHINE was following certain surgical operations. We soon had an abundant opportunity to put our principles to a practical test in regards to QUININE. It happened to be a malarial summer in Michigan. During the summer something like fifty cases came to us in all ages and in all stages of the disease. Dr. Kress and I, who could not consistently reconcile the prevailing routine QUININE PROGRAM with some of the truths we had studied, determined we would discover for ourselves what God would help us to do in malarial cases without QUININE. One member of our class was an enthusiastic advocate of QUININE. It was mutually agreed that as the patients came in, one was to be assigned to this physician, the next one to be assigned to Dr. Kress and myself, and so alternating. As he was also a microscopic expert, having taken special training in blood work, every case, not only his but ours, was carefully checked up by himself by laboratory work, so there was no chance for guesswork. It was probably as fair a test as was ever made.

We carefully took the temperature every fifteen minutes. As soon as there began to be the least rise of temperature that was a notification to us that the chill was approaching, we at once put the patient into a hot blanket pack which brought on profound perspiration, and thereby if we had hit it right we would invariably prevent the chill. The patients would perspire for a time, then we would take them out carefully, provided it was the alternate day variety we gave them tonic treatments. The following day we again instituted the temperature-taking program. We invariably found that the rise of temperature was much delayed showing that we were gaining the ascendancy. We would then go through the same program. Frequently we did not have to do this the third time. The work had been done, and in a week or ten days the patient was fully restored to health. Sometimes we would miss hitting it just right for several days, so there would be a delay.

Now for comparison: the QUININE certainly enabled the malarial patients to recover, but it was the after-history where the tremendous difference was shown. Not one of our cases had serious complications. One of the QUININE cases [of the other group] has gone through life since, practically deaf. Another one had his mentality greatly impaired, and so far as I know it has remained so to this day. Still others had minor complications.

One day an old, feeble, broken-down man came in so loaded with malaria that it seemed as though he was on the brink of the grave. According to the rotation he belonged on the QUININE LIST. The doctor, after sizing up the situation, said he did not dare to undertake this case, so he was turned over to our list. I will never forget when Dr. Kress and I went over to the Cushman Cottage, and earnestly told the Lord that His principles were on test, and pleaded with Him to vindicate what He had said. We then took hold of the case. Within a week the man was restored to health.

Melchnikoff, head of the Pasteur Institute, in his book *The New Hygiene*, says:

"It is not only OPIUM and ALCOHOL which hinder the phagocytic action. A number of other substances regularly employed in MEDICINE cause the same results. Even QUININE, the prophylactic effect of which in malarial fevers is indisputable, is a poison for the white blood cells. One should, therefore, as a general rule avoid as far as possible the use of all sorts of MEDICAMENTS, and limit oneself to the hygienic measures which may check the outbreak of infectious disease. This postulate further strengthens the thesis that the future of MEDICINE rests far more in hygiene than in therapeutics."

The remarkable work that has been done the last few years in the Tulane University, New Orleans, by one of the professors who has succeeded for the first time in cultivating malarial parasites in test tubes, outside the body, shows plainly why we are able to succeed with our packs. And he is already raising the question whether our old notion of how the QUININE killed the parasites is not erroneous; in other words, that QUININE probably only enables the body to handle the parasites just as the packs do, only in a much more expensive way to the body. If that is so, then of course that becomes one more striking commentary on that statement in the Testimonies that the use of DRUGS by our practitioners is merely a confession of their ignorance of physiology and how to use nature's remedies successfully.

Shortly after I took charge of the nervous department of the Battle Creek Sanitarium, a prominent businessman came up from Chicago. He was suffering with progressive atrophy of the left shoulder and upper arm, the muscles having already largely shrunk away. His case had been diagnosed by one of Chicago's leading neurologists who, having had his attention called to the fact that Dr. Gower in England had reported some apparent improvement in several cases by the use of STRYCHNINE INJECTIONS, recommended that he should have STRYCHNINE INJECTIONS in connection with sanitarium treatment.

I knew that the Testimonies had declared that STRYCHNINE had no business in the human body, and my conscience would not permit me to inject this as long as the man was under my care, even though an eminent physician in Chicago had ordered it to be done. I was compelled to explain to the man my conscientious scruples in regard to this, and told him that if he insisted on having this STRYCHNINE INJECTION he would have to go back to his Chicago doctor. He naturally said to me, "Will you promise to cure me with your sanitarium remedies without STRYCHNINE?" I told him "No." Progressive atrophy was considered an incurable disorder by any methods. He said he could not see the consistency of my position when the nerve specialist in Chicago had held out some hopes from STRYCHNINE, but that I did not dare to hold out positive hope with physiological remedies. I told him that I was more anxious to be right than he was to be consistent, and that I was managing my department for God. I had conscientious scruples against the use of STRYCH-NINE, and hence simply would not use it. If he wanted to have it used, it was proper to avail himself of the same, but in order to do so he would have to seek it elsewhere. He remarked that he did not know anything about my God, but did know he wanted to get well, and instead of going away he remained. In six weeks' time his muscles were fully filled in. A few years ago I dropped into the Battle Creek Sanitarium, and this man happened to be back there. He came up to me, introduced himself, and called my attention to the fact that his shoulder was all right up-to-date.

I draw no lessons from this. I am simply stating my experience, but this thing I do know, that every time we compromise we may miss a providence. Furthermore, those who compromise what they know to be principle are always in the fog, and in a little while their conscience becomes as elastic as India rubber, and it seems to be their lot and misfortune to be constantly brought into apparently impossible situations where they cannot, as far as they can see, possibly get out without further compromising principles. God never permits the man of unswerving principle to get into a situation where he considers he has any good excuse for compromising, even as much as a hair's breadth what he knows to be right.

Priessnitz, as you well know, established and maintained in Austria Silicia years ago a successful, absolutely DRUGLESS INSTITUTION. The royalty of Europe were among his patrons. Eminent men whose cases had baffled the skill of our best physicians went even from our own land to that out-of-the-way place, and were restored to health by his DRUGLESS METHODS. It was not a fad that lasted merely a year or two, but it went on year after year until it became the most notable healing center in the world. Cures were constantly being accomplished that seemed nothing short of miraculous. I have naturally been interested in that work, and I have in my library today something like twenty different books bearing on Priessnitz'work. Some of them were written by eminent physicians who themselves went there either to investigate the merits of the institution or as patients. All without exception bore testimony to the marvelous cures that this man Priessnitz secured by using nature's remedies exclusively.

The day may not be far distant when the Lord will raise up some Seventh-day Adventist Priessnitz who will effectually put to silence the lingering doubts, and the apparently unsurmountable objections to carrying out literally the program outlined for us in the Testimonies. In fact,

Appendix C

the prevailing medical practice is many days' journey nearer that ideal today than it was in Priessnitz' time. I attended the meeting of the American Medical Association a year ago in Minneapolis. My wife, Dr. Mary Paulson, attended different sections than I did so we might between us gather as many helpful facts as possible. She said that she did not hear during the time we were there a single DRUG recommended by any speaker. Dr. Cabot of Harvard was the only man who recommended a single DRUG REMEDY in my hearing, and that was large DOSES OF BISMUTH for dysentery, but he added he was not convinced that it did any good, but he knew that it could do no harm. The entire emphasis was laid upon the very remedies that the Testimonies have pointed out over and over again during these fifty years.

You raise the question of the use of ANTITOXIN in diphtheria to which I would briefly say that until I get more light than I have now, I must consider it just as natural to go to the horse for ANTITOXIN if the child is short on its own account, as it is to go to the cow for milk when the child's mother is short in this respect.

I said in the beginning of this letter that it is with much hesitancy that I write you what I am doing, for it is with a deep sense of my own shortcomings in this respect. However, that you may know that this whole matter is still a matter of conscience with me, I will enclose a copy of some correspondence that I have had just recently with a prominent physician who sent me a case of pernicious anemia with beginning of serious nerve complications. When the doctor ordered hypodermic injections of ARSENATE IRON, I tried to soothe my conscience with the fact that it was his responsibility and not mine, and that if I refrained from doing it the patient would get the same treatment at home anyway, and he would miss the sanitarium treatments which he so much needed. However, I speedily discovered that I could not make this reasoning square with my conscience, and I had to go through the humiliating experience of writing what I did, which was probably no easier for me to do than it would be for you or anyone else under similar circumstances. It is not a particularly pleasant performance to go down in the dust, although I know from previous experience that it brings the peaceable fruits of righteousness to those who are exercised thereby.

Last year we had a case of pernicious anemia here whose life hung on a thread: hemoglobin 20, and red blood cells much less than a million. I had telegraphed her husband to be here as she was about to pass away. At this juncture she whispered in Mrs. Paulson's ear, "Pray." She

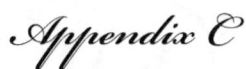

Appendix C

sent for me. We knelt down together at the woman's bedside. She was a devout woman, though not a Seventh-day Adventist. We prayed the Lord, if it pleased Him, to restore this woman to health. From that day she began to improve rapidly, and in three months' time she went home a well woman. More than a year has passed by and she is still, at the latest reports I have had, as well as ever.

I have seen such things happen too often to dare to juggle with my conscience so God would be compelled to rob me of these experiences. It is when we are in a crisis, it is when we do not know what to do next, if we endeavor to take one more step, then it is that God invariably meets us. He does not always restore our sick to health, but He gives us the signal satisfaction that we are His servants, that we have done all these things at His Word. See 1 Kings 18:36.

In *Testimonies*, vol. 9, 175, are found these significant words:

"Special instructions should be given in the art of treating the sick without the use of <u>POISONOUS </u>DRUGS, and in harmony with the light that God has given . . . they are to be educated from the standpoint of <u>conscience,</u> and as they conscientiously and faithfully follow right methods in their treatment of the sick, these methods will come to be recognized as <u>preferable</u> to the methods to which many have become accustomed, which demand the use of POISONOUS DRUGS."

How can we possibly do that unless we are willing to pay the price of having a clear-cut conscience of our own? Our nurses need to be taught that God has promised to link His blessing with the remedies that He Himself has designated rather than with those that He has condemned.

"There are many ways of practicing the healing art, but there is only one way that Heaven approves. God's remedies are the simple agencies of nature that will not tax or debilitate the system through their powerful properties." *Testimonies*, vol. 5, 443.

I fear that I have not satisfactorily answered your question. I feel humble under a sense of my own shortcomings, but I feel determined to continue to press toward the light to spell out more and more faithfully God's program.

Yours in the Master's work,

David Paulson, M.D.

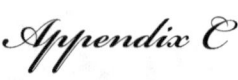

Appendix C

Appendix D

A Sketch of the Last Sickness and Death of Elder James White, (a statement by Dr. J. H. Kellogg), 18–20.

"At 8 P.M. [August 5, 1881] I examined his pulse, and remarked the same peculiarity observed the previous evening—weakness and unusual frequency, although there was no fever, neither any evidence of chill, the body being warm. He expressed himself as feeling entirely comfortable, but inclined to sleep. About five minutes later I examined his pulse again, and observed a slight irregularity. STRONG STIMULANTS were immediately administered, and Mrs. White and a number of special friends were advised that his condition was critical.

"The grave symptoms grew rapidly worse for an hour, notwithstanding the most vigorous efforts which could be made by the use of stimulating and restorative means of every sort, which were ready at hand. . . .

"At 10 A.M. [August 6, 1881] he was able to converse a little in brief sentences, but his pupils were still dilated, and the symptoms of paralysis of certain portions of the brain, which had appeared in the night, continued. . . .

"With the concurrence of the friends, we called in consultation Dr. Millspaugh of this city, whom we found in entire agreement with us in reference to the condition and the appropriate treatment. . . .

"About 1 P.M. his pulse suddenly began to increase in frequency, and soon became very feeble and irregular. Within thirty minutes he became unconscious, and his pulse rapidly rose to 176, and his respiration to 60 per minute. His temperature was 99 degrees, one-half degree above the normal temperature. The same measures used with the previous attack were again employed, but without effect, and he remained in the condition described until he breathed his last, just after 5 P.M."

Appendix E
Definition of Terms

Reference Sources:

1. *Dorland's Illustrated Medical Dictionary*, 23rd Edition, W.B. Saunders Company, 1957.

2. *Health Knowledge*—A Thorough and Concise Knowledge of the Prevention, Causes, and Treatments of Disease, Simplified for Home Use, Medical Book Distributors, Inc. 1927.

3. *Webster's New International Dictionary of the English Language*, G. and C. Merriam Company, 1916.

4. *U.S. Dispensatory 20th Ed.*, (First pub. 1877) J. B. Lippincott Co., Philadelphia 1918, p. 1818 (as per letter from Mervyn Hardinge, M.D., Ph.D., in personal file of compiler).

alterative—2. A medicine altering the processes of nutrition.

anodyne—3. Any medicine which allays pain, as an opiate or narcotic; anything that soothes disturbed feelings.

anthelmintic—1. Destructive to parasitic worms. A remedy for worms.

antiperiodic—1. Serviceable against malarial or periodic recurrence.

antisyphilitic—1. Effective against syphilis. A remedy for syphilis.

arsenate of iron—1. A chemical produced by combining arsenic with iron.

arsenic—3. One of the elements, a solid, brittle substance of tin-white to steel-grey color and metallic luster. . . . Both it and its soluble compounds are extremely poisonous, yet minute amounts of it are said to occur normally in the human body.

calomel—3. Mercurous chloride, HgCl, obtained as a fibrous, crystalline mass or a white or yellowish-white powder by subliming a mixture of metallic mercury and corrosive sublimate . . . It is heavy, insoluble, and tasteless, and is much used in medicine as a mercurial, purgative, and anthelmintic.

Appendix E

catnip—3. A well-known menthaceous plant having whorls of small blue flowers in a terminal spike. The herbage is aromatic and strong-scented, and has been used as a domestic remedy in amenorrhea, chlorosis, and flatulent colic of infants. . . . In England it is usually called *catmint*.

cholera mixture—4. The preparation contains tinctures of capsicum, rhubarb (not the garden vegetable), and opium; and spirits of camphor and peppermint, dissolved in alcohol. This was prepared by Sun. A somewhat similar preparation was prepared by Squibb.

cordial—3. Any invigorating and stimulating preparation, as a medicine, food, or drink; as, a peppermint *cordial*. Aromatized and sweetened spirit, used as a beverage; a liqueur.

decoction—1. A medicine or other substance prepared by boiling.

drug—3. Any substance used as a medicine, or in the composition of medicines, for internal or external use.

drugged liquor—Apparently any liquor to which another addictive substance such as cocaine, opium, or morphine has been added.

drugging—3. To prescribe or administer drugs or medicines.

emetic—1. Bringing on or causing the act of vomiting.

extract—1. A concentrated preparation of a vegetable or animal drug obtained by removing the active constituents therefrom with a suitable menstruum, evaporating all or nearly all the solvent, and adjusting the residual mass or powder to a prescribed standard.

febrifuge—1. A remedy that allays fever.

herb—3. A seed plant whose stem does not develop woody tissue as that of a shrub or tree, but persists only long enough for development of flowers and seeds. . . . A plant of economic value; specifically, one used for medicinal purposes, or for its sweet scent or flavor.

hop—3. A twining, moraceous vine with 3-lobed or 5-lobed leaves and small, greenish, diclinous flowers, the pistillate growing in cones or strobiles known as "hops" for which the plant is commonly cultivated. The ripened and dried pistillate cones of this plant are used chiefly to impart a bitter flavor to malt liquors, and also in medicine as a tonic and soporific.

Appendix E

infusion—1. The product of the process of steeping a drug for the extraction of its medicinal principles.

intoxicate—3. To poison. To make drunk; to inebriate; to excite or to stupefy by strong drink or by a narcotic substance. To excite to a trans- port of enthusiasm, frenzy, or madness; to elate unduly or excessively.

liquor—3. Specifically, an alcoholic beverage, as brandy, wine, whiskey, beer, etc.;—often limited to such as are strong or distilled; as, beer, wines, and *liquors*.

Liquor, poisonous—See drugged liquor.

medicinal—3. Curative or alleviative; used for the cure or alleviation of bodily disorders; as, *medicinal* tinctures, plants, or springs.

medicine—3. Any substance or preparation used in treating disease; a medicament; a remedial agent; a remedy; physic.

mercury—3. A heavy, silver-white, liquid, metallic element;—called also, popularly, *quicksilver*. Mercury occurs native, and in cinnabar, calomel, and a few other minerals. It is chiefly prepared by roasting cinnabar and condensing the vapors. It is the only metal that is liquid at ordinary temperatures. . . . Its compounds are used in medicine as purgatives, alteratives, and especially as antisyphilitics. Its alloys are called amalgams. The element and its compounds are poisonous.

morphine—3. A bitter, white, crystalline, narcotic base, the principal alkaloid of opium. It is found also in some other plants besides the opium poppy, as *Argemone mexicana* and *Humulus lupulus* (wild hops). It is like opium in medical properties, though less stimulating and constipating, and is used as an anodyne and soporific.

mustard—3. Any brassicaceous plant of the genus *Sinapis*, generally recognizable by the lyrately-lobed leaves, yellow flowers, and linear beaked pods. . . . A sharp pungent powder composed of ground mustard seed, . . . which is made into a paste by mixing with water, etc., for use as a condiment and as a rubefacient or counterirritant. . . . Mustard is a stimulant and diuretic, and in large doses an emetic.

narcotic—3. A drug which in moderate doses allays susceptibility, relieves pain, and produces profound sleep, but which in poisonous doses produces stuper, coma, or convulsions. The chief narcotics are opium (with morphine), belladonna (with atropine), Indian hemp,

Appendix E

stramonium, hyoscyamus, and lactucarium.

nostrum—3. A medicine recommended by its preparer; especially, a medicine the ingredients of which are kept secret by the inventor or proprietor; a patent medicine; a quack medicine.

noxious—3. Hurtful; harmful; baneful; pernicious; injurious; destructive; unwholesome; insalubrious.

nux vomica—3. The poisonous seed of an Asiatic loganiaceous tree. It contains several alkaloids, chiefly strychnine, and brucine.

opiate—3. Any medicine containing, or derived from, opium, and tending to induce sleep or repose; a narcotic. Anything which induces rest or inaction; that which quiets uneasiness.

opium—3. A drug consisting of the inspissated juice of the opium poppy. It is obtained from incisions made in the capsules of the plant, the best flowing from the first incision. . . . It is of a brownish-yellow color, has a faint smell, and bitter, acrid taste. It is a stimulant, narcotic poison which may produce hallucinations, profound sleep, or death. It is much used in medicine to soothe pain and inflammation, and is smoked as an intoxicant with baneful effects. In addition to the gum, wax, and minor compounds constituting over 75 per cent of its weight, opium contains about 20 different alkaloids, the chief of which is morphine.

patent medicine—1. Vernacular term for a nostrum advertised to the public. It is generally of secret composition.

pernicious—3. Having the quality of injuring or killing; destructive; fatal; ruinous; very mischievous; as, *pernicious* to health.

poison—3. Any agent which introduced into the animal organism may produce a morbid, noxious, or deadly effect.

poisonous drinks—See drugged liquors.

poultice—3. A soft composition, as of bread, bran, herbs, or the like, usually heated and spread on a cloth, to be applied to sores, inflamed parts of the body, etc., to supply warmth, or moisture, or act as an anodyne, emollient, antiseptic, counterirritant, etc.; a cataplasm.

purgative—2. A medicine producing copious evacuations.

quinine—3. An alkaloid extracted from the bark of various species of *Cinchona* as a bitter white crystalline substance . . . employed as a febrifuge or antiperiodic.

rubefacient—1. An agent that reddens the skin by producing active or passive hyperemia (increased blood flow).

sarsaparilla—3. Any of various Mexican, Central American, or South American species of *Smilax*, as *S. officinalis, S. papyracea,* and *S. medica.* The dried, cordlike roots of any of these. It is used in the form of a decoction, infusion, fluid extract, or syrup, as a mild tonic and alterative.

smartweed—3. The water pepper (*Polygonum hydropiper*); also, any of several other species of *Polygonum* having acrid juice.

soporific—1. Causing or inducing profound sleep. A drug or other agent which induces sleep.

spirit—3. In the old chemistry, any liquid produced by distillation; in modern use, any strong distilled alcoholic liquor; especially, ordinary, or ethyl, alcohol. . . . A solution in alcohol of a volatile principle; tincture.

spirituous—3. Containing, or of the nature of, alcoholic spirit; alcoholic.

squill—3. A bulbous, liliaceous plant of southern Europe sometimes grown in gardens for its long racemes of small white flowers. The bulb of this plant is cut in thin slices for use as an expectorant and diuretic. In large doses it is emetic and purgative.

stimulant—3. That which stimulates, provokes, or excites; . . . an agent which produces a temporary increase of vital activity in the organism, or in any of its parts; sometimes, specifically, an alcoholic beverage.

strychnine—3. A very poisonous alkaloid obtained from various species of plants, especially of the genus *Strychnos*, as from the seeds of the St. Ignatius' bean and from nux vomica. It is a white, crystalline substance, having a very bitter, acrid taste, and is employed in medicine as a powerful neurotic stimulant and also for its tonic action on the heart.

tonic—3. Increasing strength or tone in the system; obviating the effects of debility and restoring healthy functions.

Appendix E

Home and
...Health...

A HOUSEHOLD MANUAL

CONTAINING TWO THOUSAND
RECIPES AND HELPFUL SUGGES-
TIONS ON THE BUILDING AND
CARE OF THE HOME IN HAR-
MONY WITH SANITARY LAWS;
THE PRESERVATION OF HEALTH
BY CLEAN, CONSISTENT LIVING;
AND THE HOME TREATMENT OF
THE MORE SIMPLE AILMENTS
AND DISEASES, BY THE USE OF
NATURAL, RATIONAL REME-
DIES INSTEAD OF DRUGS

PREPARED AND
EDITED BY A
COMPETENT
COMMITTEE OF
HOME-MAKERS
AND PHYSICIANS

Pacific Press Publishing Co.

Mountain View, California

Portland, Ore.   Kansas City, Mo.

1907

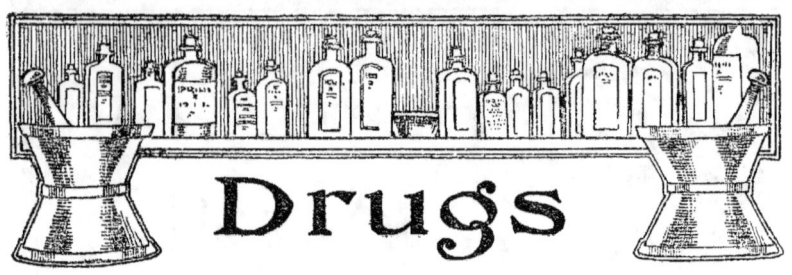

Drugs

A POISONED SYSTEM

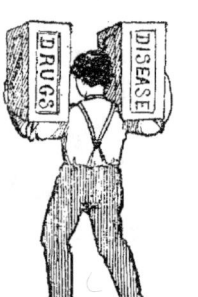

A Heavy Load

Disease, in most cases, is the result of accumulated poisons in the system. A diseased condition may be compared to a ship with a heavy list to one side. How shall the ship be righted? There are two ways. A portion of the cargo may be removed from the heavily weighted side, or additional cargo may be put aboard to balance up the load. One method lightens the load, and the other increases it. By continuing to increase the cargo in this way whenever there is a list to one side, the ship is endangered, and may go to the bottom in the first great storm.

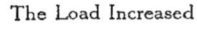

The Load Increased

LIGHTEN THE LOAD

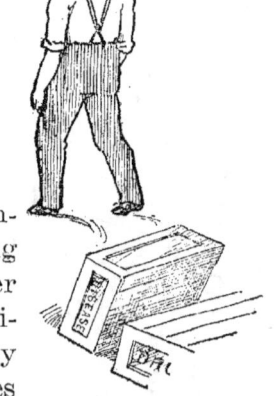

The Load Removed

When a man is sick, his body is generally loaded with poisons. In seeking relief he should first consider whether he will increase the load by taking poisonous drugs, or lighten the load by eliminating the poisons. If he takes additional poison into his system, he may find temporary relief, and continue to sail the sea of

[515]

Appendix F

" The blessed, heaven-sent water, skilfully applied, would quench the hot fever, but it is set aside for poisonous drugs."

---

life as long as the weather is fair, but when the storm breaks upon him, the chances are that he will go down.

THE AMERICAN DRUG CURSE

"The disastrous and damning consequences of this curse to America," writes J. R. Stevenson, in *Physical Culture,* "are hardly known or appreciated by the public. The citizens of our country have been accustomed to seeing the ever-present saloon and drug-store till they look upon them almost as necessary parts of our civilization. They have had so many agents at work in their favor, and ignorance of the things that pertain to and promulgate physical health is so general and dense, that to the thinking man or woman it is little wonder that these dens are so numerous, or that their victims are such a multitude.

"The most noteworthy thing about America that impresses one who travels far over its fertile territory, is the enormous number of physical wrecks encountered—thin, emaciated, pale-faced men and women, who face you at every turn; who come into your offices, or sit beside you in the cars, and appear to be dragging out an aimless existence."

Mr. Stevenson states a truth too well known in America when he attributes a large share of this physical weakness to the effects of powerful drugs and patent medicines. America has become a fair field for the manufacture and sale of such powerful nostrums. As our population has rapidly increased, "drug venders and their victims have increased proportionately. The drug-store and the saloon keep close pace with the pioneers in the so-called march of progress."

"Science has endeavored to show that certain drugs are poisonous, that they produce evil effects upon organs and tissues when mixed with the elements of any living

Appendix F

" The usual custom of annihilating pain by some powerful drug is a most unnatural practice."

organism; yet, under one disguise or another, nearly all
of these potent factors of physical degeneration are sold
publicly and under the protection of our liberal government."

A HIGHROAD TO INTEMPERANCE

There is no surer pathway to intemperance than that
which is entered through the gateway of patent medicines,
and these gateways are kept open by the permission of
our government, and its porters are licensed and pro-
tected by law. Patent medicines are dangerous chiefly because of the large per cent of alcohol and opium which
they contain.

In an editorial in *American Medicine,* this question is
asked, "Why do not the temperance people fight the patent-
medicine enemy?" And again, "If it is admitted that the
army canteen made drunkards, surely the patent-medicine
syndicates make a thousand times as many. No one is
ignorant of the fact that there are many million dollars'
worth of these alcoholic nostrums sold each year, and that
multitudes of people are thus secretly and ignorantly
turned into drunkards. Doctor Bumgardner, in 'Transactions Colorado State Medical Society for 1902,' says that
the following patent medicines contain the percentage given
of alcohol:—

Green's Nervura	17.2
Hood's Sarsaparilla	18.8
Schenck's Seaweed Tonic	19.5
Brown's Iron Bitters	19.7
Kaufman's Sulphur Bitters	20.5
Paine's Celery Compound	21.0
Burdock's Blood Bitters	25.2
Ayers' Sarsaparilla	26.2
Warner's Safe Tonic Bitters	35.7
Parker's Tonic	41.6
Hostetter's Stomach Bitters	44.3

Appendix F

Drugs undoubtedly bring relief, but only by paralyzing the nerves.—A. B. Olson, M. D.

Dr. Ashbel P. Grinnell, of New York City, after making a statistical study of patent medicines, vouches for the truthfulness of the statement "that more alcohol is consumed in this country in patent medicines than is dispensed in a legal way by licensed liquor venders, barring the sales of ales and beer."

Statistics from the official reports of the Massachusetts State Board of Health, concerning such remedies as Hood's Sarsaparilla, Ayers' Sarsaparilla, Liebig Company's Cocoa-Beef Tonic, Parker's Beef Tonic, Boker's Stomach Bitters, and Warner's Safe Tonic Bitters, are as follows:—

"Ordinary whisky, as dispensed in saloons, is scarcely stronger in alcoholic content than are most of these so-called remedies, and especially some of them that are recommended for the treatment of inebriates and the alcoholic habit. . . . It is very probable that at the present moment the temperance societies of this country could do nothing better calculated to advance the cause of temperance than to undertake a vigorous crusade against the use of such remedies."

OPIUM AND COCAINE

Although it is well known that opium and cocaine are the most enslaving and body and soul destroying of all drugs, and although drugs are the most active agents for making slaves to these evils, yet "our drug makers and venders hold forth these poisons, to an ignorant and credulous populace, in many disguised forms, as a panacea for all ills. As patent soothing syrups, colic conquerors, and pain killers, it is retailed in small bottles to anxious mothers for doctoring their children. Even the family physician, when called in to prescribe for a tiny stomach that has been overloaded, writes hieroglyphics, which, when presented to the ubiquitous druggist, call for a preparation in

Appendix F

Drugs   519

Drugs give relief only temporarily and the last state of
the patient is often worse than the first.

---

which this damnable pain killer, nerve wrecker, tissue
destroyer, is the prominent ingredient; and the little stomach takes in the poison, to deaden the nerves and disturb
organic functions, and shock all the forces of life.

"All its ill effects no man can trace; how many infants
are hidden away underground, year after year, the victims
of their own loving mothers' misguided solicitude, and this
deadly agent of the doctor and drug vender, no man can
ever number."—*J. R. Stevenson*

PAREGORIC

"Doctors vary in their opinion," says Maud Banfield
in an able article in the *Ladies' Home Journal,* "as to
whether opium, alcohol, or cocaine is the most generally
harmful constituent in the greater number of patent medicines and 'cures.' One reads of 'paregoric habits' which
are 'cured' by a medicine bearing a fair-sounding name,
which, upon analysis, is found to contain several times the
quantity of opium existing in the paregoric mixture. A
great many people seem to think that paregoric is a harmless, soothing mixture, good to give the baby when he cries,
or just the thing for Johnie when he suffers the consequences of eating an unsuitable number of green apples.
The Latin name for paregoric is *tinctura opii camphorata,*
or camphorated tincture of opium. One ounce, or two table-
spoonfuls, of the mixture contains two grains of opium.
It is more constipating that the other preparations of
opium, owing to the camphor.

"The stomach-ache from which Johnie suffers in consequence of too many green apples or too much pie, is
nature's warning signal—it is a symptom, not a disease.
If you saw a red light on a railway track warning another
train that there was danger ahead, you would not think
you removed the danger if you merely removed the red

Appendix F

Most patent medicines contain a large percentage of alcohol. Their effects are deceptive and they lead to intemperance.

light. The cause of this stomach-ache must be removed, and a dose of castor-oil or salts in proper quantities, which would help clear nature's track, is surely greater common sense than quieting the warning signal. Pain is always a symptom—never a disease.

"If the baby cries, and you are convinced that he cries because he suffers, you must try to arrive at and remove the cause—not give him a 'soothing syrup,' which may give both you and the baby a quiet half-hour at the cost of life itself."

DANGEROUS POWDERS

Under this head may be mentioned a large variety of powders and tablets recommended as a cure for headache, catarrh, depression, etc. In placing these goods upon the market, they are represented as containing a harmless combination of mild ingredients, whereas their supposed virtue lies chiefly in the presence, in dangerous quantities, of such powerful and demoralizing poisons as cocaine, opium, or acetanilide. These are the worst sort of patent medicines, the most deceptive in their character, and the most deadly in their effects.

BETTER REMEDIES

Drug medication is a curse. Within our reach are better remedies than these. "Nature will respond to God's remedies." Pure air, pure water, exercise, rest, and many other natural curative agencies are within our reach. We need only to become intelligent as to their proper use, and the harmful drugs may be set aside.

Appendix F

Appendix G
Many treatments in this chapter are not safe.

[See introductory remarks on page 6.]

HEALTH KNOWLEDGE

A THOROUGH AND CONCISE KNOWLEDGE OF
THE PREVENTION, CAUSES, AND TREATMENTS
OF DISEASE, SIMPLIFIED FOR HOME USE

THIRTY-FOUR DEPARTMENTS
INCLUDING

PRENATAL CARE AND THE CARE OF INFANTS, HEALTH IN CHILDHOOD, PREG-
NANCY AND MOTHERHOOD, WOMEN'S PHYSICAL CHANGES AND THEIR
DISORDERS, DISEASES OF WOMEN, PHYSICAL CULTURE AND DEEP-
BREATHING EXERCISES FOR MEN AND WOMEN, PHYSICAL
CULTURE AND MASSAGE FOR INFANTS, FOODS AND
THEIR VALUES, HOME NURSING, HOME REME-
DIES, MEDICAL PRESCRIPTIONS IN LATIN
AND ENGLISH, PLANTS, VEGE-
TABLES, FRUITS, HERBS

EDITOR-IN-CHIEF
J. L. CORISH, M. D.

FORMERLY ASSOCIATED WITH THE BROOKLYN EASTERN DISTRICT HOSPITAL;
MANHATTAN EYE AND EAR HOSPITAL, NEW YORK CITY; MEDICAL SUPT.
OF THE NEW YORK STATE HOME AT FORT HAMILTON, N. Y.

ASSISTED BY A CORPS OF COMPETENT PHYSI-
CIANS AND SURGEONS FROM THE LEADING
HOSPITALS, COLLEGES AND UNIVERSITIES OF
THE UNITED STATES AND FOREIGN COUNTRIES

VOLUME II

MEDICAL BOOK DISTRIBUTORS, Inc.

PUBLISHERS
NEW YORK
1927

Many treatments in this chapter are not safe.

COUGH

In the great majority of instances cough is due to something wrong in the respiratory system—larynx, windpipe, bronchial tubes, or lungs—sometimes to conditions outside the respiratory organs. A dry cough, with little or no expectoration, occurs in the first stages of bronchitis, consumption, asthma, whooping-cough, influenza, and pneumonia; also in pleurisy; inhalation of dust or irritating fumes; or from the tickling of a long uvula. A single, slight, dry cough, frequently repeated, is the "hacking" cough of the earliest stages of consumption.

A loose cough with abundant expectoration occurs in the later stages of the diseases first mentioned above, and in some other lung diseases.

Cough coming in fits or paroxysms is seen most characteristically in whooping-cough. A paroxysmal cough with long intervals between may be due to cavities in the lung. Under such circumstances large amounts are expectorated in a short time, the cough ceasing until the cavity fills up again.

Laryngeal Cough.—This is dry but hoarse, ringing or "brassy" in character. It may be due to laryngitis, croup, or to food particles going in "the wrong way." The monotonous croaking cough sometimes due to hysteria is also laryngeal, and so is the cough met with in some cases of aneurism of the aorta.

Suppressed cough is a sign that coughing is painful or exhausting, as in pneumonia, pleurisy, and peritonitis.

Winter cough, disappearing in summer, means either chronic bronchitis or a very chronic form of consumption.

Cough due to conditions outside the respiratory organs may come from hysteria, wax in the ear, adenoids, long uvula, aneurism, or heart disease.

Stomach cough is found at times in the subjects of chronic gastric catarrh.

The treatment of cough depends on the cause, for intelligent treatment should be directed toward removing the cause and not merely suppressing the cough. If very incessant and troublesome, sedative drugs may be necessary; but it is by no means always safe to check cough by these means, especially in children

Appendix G

Many treatments in this chapter are not safe.

722   DISEASES OF THE RESPIRATORY ORGANS

and old people.   We would merely say that in the great majority of cases great relief is given to a cough if the air inhaled be moist. This can be accomplished by having a kettle with a long spout projecting into the room, or by inhaling occasionally the steam coming from a pitcher of boiling water.

The following are well used formulas for different ages:

OLD FOLKS

℞   Aromatic Spirits of Ammonia ....one fluid ounce
Spirits of Chloroform ....two fluid drams
Peppermint-water ....two fluid ounces
Mix.
DOSE: One teaspoonful every four hours.

CHILDREN

℞   Wine of Ipecac ....one fluid dram
Brown Mixture modified without
Opium ....four fluid ounces
Mix.
DOSE: Ten to fifteen drops in water every four hours.

INFANTS

℞   Spirits of Camphor ....five minims
Tincture of Belladonna ....two minims
Quinine Sulphate ....three grains
Syrup Tolu ....three fluid ounces
Mix.
DOSE: One-half teaspoonful every three hours.

FROM 16 TO 50 YEARS OLD

℞   Syrup of Tolu ......four fluid drams
Syrup of Squill ......one and one-half fluid ounces
Wine of Ipecac ......one and one-half fluid ounces
Brown Mixture modified without
Opium ....two and one-half fluid ounces
Mix.
DOSE: One teaspoonful every three hours.

Or:

℞   White Pine and Tar Syrup ......four fluid ounces
DOSE: One teaspoonful every three hours.

Appendix G

Many treatments in this chapter are not safe.

Immediate relief is best assured by local treatment, and the following is a favorite formula:

R Menthol ....one grain
   Camphor ....one grain
   Liquid Petroleum ....one ounce
Mix.

DIRECTIONS: Place two drops on a piece of cotton and insert into each nostril.

Or:

R Liquid Peptonoids and Creosote ..four fluid ounces
DOSE: One teaspoonful every three hours.

Or:

R Chloride of Ammonia ..two drams
   Fluidextract of Licorice.two fluid drams
   Syrup of Wild Cherry ..one fluid ounce
   Water ....one and one-half fluid ounces
Mix.

DOSE: One teaspoonful every three hours.

HICCOUGH

Definition.—Hiccough is a spasmodic indrawing of air to the lungs, ending with a click, due to sudden closure of the vocal cords. The cause is some irritation of the nerves which go to the diaphragm, producing sudden contractions of the latter. Most cases, especially those recurring habitually about the same hour of the day, are due to indigestion, and the symptom also occurs in some serious general diseases, like the uremia of Bright's disease and typhoid fever, being in such cases a grave sign.

Treatment.—If the condition be due to dyspepsia, it is often relieved by some aromatic like a teaspoonful of Hoffmann's anodyne, or a tablespoonful of peppermint water or cinnamon water. When continuous and excessive it is usually controlled by bromides.

R Ammonium Bromide ....six teaspoonfuls
   Spirits of Anise ....twenty drops
   Simple Elixir ....two ounces
DOSE: One teaspoonful, when the attack starts.

Appendix G

Many treatments in this chapter are not safe.

724   DISEASES OF THE RESPIRATORY ORGANS

One teaspoonful of vinegar mixed with one teaspoonful of sugar and eaten slowly will often relieve.

Taking nine sips of water and at the same time holding the breath will often prove effective.

Simple methods have proved very successful when all other methods and medication have been tried. The most noted (both of which were discovered by accident in endeavoring to accomplish other treatment and which have since never failed) are: (1) Press the back of the tongue down and backward with the handle of a large spoon for about one minute. This is to be continued if the hiccough returns, as it generally does, when, after two or three treatments, it will cease for good. (2) This method (one which is praised the most) is to stretch the tongue by holding it between the fingers or a suitable instrument, as tongue forceps, pulling it out as far as possible and holding it there for two minutes.

A simple and effective remedy is:

    ℞   Tincture of Camphor ....three drops
         Ammonia-water (medicinal) ....three drops
  DIRECTIONS: Add to one-half glass of water.

When due to indigestion, the following is recommended:
    ℞   Bicarbonate of Soda ....one dram
         Tincture of Nux Vomica ....one dram
         Tincture of Cardamom ....three ounces
  DOSE: One teaspoonful in water before meals.

BREATHLESSNESS

Pleurisy causes short, rapid breathing to avoid the pain of deep inspiration.

Narrowing of the air-passages may produce sudden and alarming attacks of difficult breathing, especially among children; e.g., in laryngismus, croup, asthma and diphtheria (see these headings).

Almost all *affections of the heart* cause breathlessness when the person undergoes any special exertion.

Among the *general diseases* which may interfere with breathing, the uremia of Bright's disease and the coma at the end of diabetes must be noted.

Appendix G

Many treatments in this chapter are not safe.

MEDICINES WITH THEIR USES AND DOSES

The various medicines with their individual uses and properties, also their doses, which are approximate, are here given. No definite dosage is applicable to all cases, as some individuals are more readily affected by certain drugs than others; and, moreover, the age of the patient is to be considered.

Ordinarily, the following doses are prescribed for adults; proportionate doses for children are given in the Table of Weights and Measures on pages 551 and 552.

DRUG	PROPERTIES AND USES	DOSE
Acacia, powder.......	Demulcent; expectorant	30 grains when necessary.
Aconite, tincture......	Sedative; narcotic; reduces fever.......	1 to 5 drops three times a day.
Aloes, powdered......	Ecbolic; purgative....	3 to 5 grains at night.
Aloes and Myrrh, pills	Ecbolic; stimulant....	2 pills three times a day.
Alum, powder.......	Emetic; astringent....	3 to 30 grains twice a day.
Alum, burnt, powder..	Escharotic	15 grains, moistened, applied once a day.
Ammonia, Aromatic Spirits	Stimulant	½ teaspoonful every three hours.
Ammonia-water	Caustic; stimulant....	10 drops in water three times a day.
Ammonium Benzoate, powder	Antirheumatic	15 grains every three hours.
Ammonium Bromide, powder	Depressant	20 grains three times a day.
Ammonium Carbonate, powder	Stimulant	3 to 5 grains every four hours.
Ammonium Chloride, powder	Expectorant	5 grains every four hours.
Ammonium Iodide, powder	Alterative	4 grain three times a day.
Ammonium Salicylate, powder	Antirheumatic	5 grains every four hours.

1263

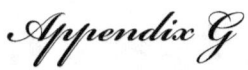
Appendix G

Many treatments in this chapter are not safe.

1264   PHARMACEUTICAL

DRUG	PROPERTIES AND USES	DOSE
Amyl Nitrite, liquid..	Motor-depressant	3 drops every four hours.
Angelica-root, fluid-extract	Stimulant	1 teaspoonful three times a day.
Aniseed, essence......	Aromatic; carminative	1 teaspoonful once a day.
Antimony, wine......	Emetic; expectorant..	15 drops three times a day.
Antipyrine, powder...	Analgesic	3 grains every four hours.
Apocynum, fluid-extract	Expectorant	10 drops every three hours.
Arrowroot, powder....	Tonic; nutritive......	4 tablespoonfuls twice a day.
Arsenic, Fowler's Solution	Alterative	1 drop three times a day.
Arsenous Acid, powder	Stimulant	1/60 grain three times a day.
Arsenous Iodide, powder	Digestive	1/30 grain three times a day.
Asafetida, powder....	Cathartic; antiseptic..	3 grains every four hours.
Atropina, powder....	Narcotic; anodyne....	1/200 grain three times a day.
Balsam Copaiba, liquid	Diuretic; laxative....	20 drops three times a day.
Balsam Fir, liquid....	Diuretic	10 drops every four hours.
Balsam Peru, liquid...	Stimulant; tonic......	10 drops three times a day.
Balsam Tolu, tincture.	Antiseptic; expectorant	20 drops every three hours.
Belladonna, tincture..	Narcotic; anodyne....	3 drops three times a day.
Benzoic Acid, powder.	Diuretic	5 grains every three hours.
Berberis, powder.....	Tonic; stimulant.....	25 grains three times a day.
Betanaphthol, powder.	Antiseptic	2 grains every three hours.
Bismuth Ammonium Citrate, powder.....	Astringent	2 grains three times a day.
Bismuth Subcarbonate, powder	Astringent	5 grains every four hours.
Bismuth Subnitrate, powder	Sedative	10 grains three times a day.

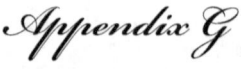

Appendix G

Many treatments in this chapter are not safe.

MEDICINES WITH THEIR USES AND DOSES   1265

DRUG	PROPERTIES AND USES	DOSE
Bittersweet, fluid-extract	Emetic	30 drops three times a day.
Blackberry, cordial	Aromatic; carminative	2 tablespoonfuls every six hours.
Black Cohosh, infusion	Narcotic; diuretic	1 wineglassful three times a day.
Blue Mass, pills	Alterative; cathartic	2 pills at night.
Blue Vitriol, powder	Emetic	1 grain three times a day.
Boneset, infusion	Stimulant	1 tablespoonful three times a day.
Borax, powder	Detergent	15 grains every four hours.
Bromoform, liquid	Sedative	3 drops three times a day.
Bryonia, fluidextract	Irritant	8 drops every six hours.
Buchu, infusion	Diuretic	1 tablespoonful every three hours.
Buckthorn, fluid-extract	Cathartic	1 teaspoonful at night.
Burdock, fluidextract	Herpetic	1 tablespoonful three times a day.
Caffeine, powder	Cerebral stimulant	1 grain every four hours.
Calamus, fluidextract	Aromatic	10 drops after meals.
Calcium Carbonate, powder	Antacid	10 grains three times a day.
Calcium Hypophosphite, powder	Tonic	5 grains every four hours.
Calomel, powder	Cathartic; antiseptic	2 to 5 grains at one dose.
Calumba, decoction	Tonic	1 tablespoonful three times a day.
Calumba, fluidextract	Stomachic	20 grains after meals.
Camphor, powder	Antiseptic; cathartic	2 to 5 grains every three hours.
Camphor, Monobromated, powder	Sedative	1 grain every four hours.
Camphoric Acid, powder	Night-sweats	15 grains at night.
Cannabis Indica, fluidextract	Narcotic	1 drop three times a day.
Cantharis, tincture	Diuretic; stimulant	3 drops twice a day.
Capsicum, tincture	Carminative	5 drops after meals.

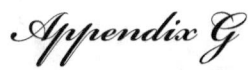

Appendix G

Many treatments in this chapter are not safe.

1270 PHARMACEUTICAL

DRUG	PROPERTIES AND USES	DOSE
Lithium Salicylate, powder	Antiarthritic	15 grains three times a day.
Lobelia, tincture	Diuretic	30 drops every four hours.
Lupulinum, powder	Narcotic	5 grains three times a day.
Magnesium, powder	Antacid	30 grains after meals.
Magnesium Carbonate, powder	Laxative	1 teaspoonful twice a day.
Manganese Sulphate, powder	Alterative	4 grains three times a day.
Mastic, gum	Stomachic	20 grains three times a day.
Matico, powder	Aromatic	30 grains after meals.
Mercuric Yellow Iodide, powder	Alterative	1/10 grain three times a day.
Mercury Bichloride	Antiseptic	1/20 grain three times a day.
Mercury with chalk	Intestinal antiseptic	4 grains every four hours.
Morphine, powder	Narcotic	¼ grain when necessary.
Moschus, powder	Stimulant	4 grains three times a day.
Myrrh, gum	Carminative	5 grains every four hours.
Naphthaline, crystals	Antiseptic	1 grain every three hours.
Nitric Acid, dilute	Stimulant	20 drops before meals.
Nux Vomica, tincture	Stomachic	5 drops after meals.
Opium, tincture	Narcotic	10 drops when needed.
Oxgall, purified	Digestive	5 grains after meals.
Pancreatine, powder	Digestive	5 grains before meals.
Paraldehyde, liquid	Hypnotic	30 drops every four hours.
Paregoric, liquid	Sedative	15 drops every four hours.
Pareira, powder	Alterative	20 grains three times a day.
Pelletierine, powder	Teniafuge	2 grains every four hours.
Pepo, emulsion	Teniafuge	1 ounce at night.
Peppermint-water	Carminative	1 ounce after meals.

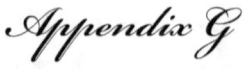

Appendix G

Many treatments in this chapter are not safe.

MEDICINES WITH THEIR USES AND DOSES   1271

DRUG	PROPERTIES AND USES	DOSE
Pepsine, powder	Digestive	2 grains every four hours.
Phenacetine, powder	Analgesic	5 grains every six hours.
Phosphoric Acid, dilute	Stomachic	10 drops before each meal.
Phosphorus Elixir	Nerve stimulant	1 teaspoonful three times a day.
Physostigma, powder	Antineuralgic	½ grain three times a day.
Phytolacca, powder	Alterative	8 grains every four hours.
Pilocarpine, powder	Diuretic	1/10 grain every six hours.
Pine Tar, syrup	Expectorant	1 teaspoonful every three hours.
Piperina, powder	Antiperiodic	1 grain three times a day.
Podophyllum, powder	Cholagogue	5 grains at night.
Potassium Acetate, powder	Alterative	15 grains after meals.
Potassium Bicarbonate, powder	Diuretic	20 grains every four hours.
Potassium Bromide, powder	Nerve sedative	10 grains every three hours.
Potassium Chlorate, powder	Astringent	4 grains every four hours.
Potassium Citrate, crystals	Refrigerant	15 grains three times a day.
Potassium Cyanide, crystals	Cough sedative	1/20 grain every three hours.
Potassium Hypophosphite, crystals	Nerve tonic	5 grains after meals.
Potassium Iodide, crystals	Alterative	5 grains three times a day.
Potassium Permanganate, crystals	Deodorant	½ grain every four hours.
Potassium Sulphate, crystals	Cathartic	15 grains every three hours.
Quinine Sulphate, powder	Antiperiodic	4 grains every two hours.
Resorcin, powder	Antiseptic	1 grain every six hours.
Rheum, powder	Cathartic	10 grains three times a day.
Rhus Glabra, powder	Astringent	10 grains every three hours.

Appendix G

Many treatments in this chapter are not safe.

1272   PHARMACEUTICAL

DRUG	PROPERTIES AND USES	DOSE
Rubus, powder.......	Tonic	15 grains after meals.
Rubus Glabra, powder.	Refrigerant	10 grains three times a day.
Sabal, powder........	Diuretic	10 grains every three hours.
Salicylic Acid, powder	Antirheumatic	5 grains every four hours.
Salol, powder........	Analgesic	5 grains every four hours.
Saltpeter, powder.....	Antiseptic	7 grains every six hours.
Sanguinaria, powder..	Expectorant	1 grain three times a day.
Santonine, powder....	Anthelmintic	1 grain each night.
Sarsaparilla, syrup...	Alterative	1 tablespoonful after meals.
Senega, fluidextract...	Expectorant	10 grains three times a day.
Senna, powder.......	Cathartic	1 teaspoonful at night.
Sodium Benzoate, powder	Antipyretic	10 grains every four hours.
Sodium Bromide, powder	Nerve sedative........	15 grains every three hours.
Sodium Citrate, powder	Diuretic	15 grains three times a day.
Sodium Salicylate, powder	Antineuralgic	10 grains every four hours.
Sparteine, powder....	Cardiac stimulant.....	1/5 grain three times a day.
Spigelia, powder......	Vermifuge	1 teaspoonful after meals.
Squill, powder........	Expectorant	1 grain every four hours.
Stillingia, powder.....	Alterative	15 grains three times a day.
Stramonium, powder..	Analgesic	1 grain every four hours.
Strontium Bromide, powder	Sedative	10 grains every four hours.
Strontium Iodide, powder	Alterative	5 grains three times a day.
Strontium Salicylate, powder	Antiseptic	15 grains four times a day.
Strychnine, powder...	Stimulant	1/60 grain after meals.
Styrax, gum.........	Alterative	10 grains three times a day.

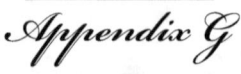

Appendix G

Appendix H
Treating Fire With Fire

"A Case of Total Blindness; Possibly Due to an Overdose of Quinin," *JAMA*. 1896; 27:992, as quoted in *Journal of the American Medical Association*, November 6, 1996—Vol 276, No. 17, 1364.

August 8, 1895, I was called to J. W., a man 34 years old. After repeated questioning of the patient and his sister, the following disconnected, incomplete and probably somewhat inaccurate history was elicited: The young man was an accountant in the employ of one of the Texas railroads and had been with them for years, although for some time he had been an OPIUM, WHISKEY and TOBACCO HABITUÉ. The first habit he had contracted as a result of the use of OPIUM during an attack of dysentery. Four years ago, he had gone to an institute and had been cured of these habits, but quickly lapsed into them again, excepting that he never renewed the use of TOBACCO.

I was unable to find out definitely the amount of MORPHINE and WHISKEY that he used daily. His own statement was to the effect that he had been taking about 7 grains of MORPHINE daily. This statement was probably inaccurate, for judging from the amount it was necessary to give to keep him reasonably quiet, at the time I was called, he certainly could not have been taking less than from 10 to 20 grains in the twenty-four hours, and probably more for some months; and of WHISKEY he used from one pint to one quart daily.

In October, 1894, when suffering from malaria, he had been given by a physician 120 grains of QUININE in twenty-four hours in four doses. In a very short time he was totally blind in both eyes, but this condition lasted only about two weeks, after which there was a gradual return of vision, so that he resumed work on his books, and was able to continue at intervals by aid of an assistant (for his vision never became good), till February, 1895, since which time he had not been able to see anything, except to distinguish a bright light occasionally. There was no history of concurrent deafness.

During June and July he had been living with a woman who was an OPIUM HABITUÉ, and she had kept him constantly saturated with MORPHINE till his sister brought him to Los Angeles.

The patient, five feet nine or ten inches tall, was extremely emaciated, weighing about 103 pounds: his normal weight had been from 145 to 150. He had the marked OPIUM CACHEXIA [wasting] and puffiness of the lower lids. There was almost complete loss of cutaneous and deep reflexes, the knee jerk being entirely absent. The bowels were sluggish, and the urine very scanty, ten to twelve ounces in twenty-four hours. He was practically demented, his memory so defective that he could not sustain a conversation.

The pupils were so small that it was quite impossible in his helpless condition to make a satisfactory ophthalmoscopic examination without producing mydriasis [pupil dilation], which I did with a weak solution of SULPHATE OF ATROPINE, and found the fundi presenting very small deviations from the normal. Both nerves were pallid and the arteries and veins, though relatively normal, were both slightly reduced in size, no other changes could be detected.

The MORPHINE was gradually diminished and CODEINE substituted, the WHISKEY slowly reduced, so that by November 1, he was taking no MORPHINE or WHISKEY.

At different times, TRIONAL in 15 grain doses, CHLORALAMID 30 grains, CHLORAL and BROMIDS 20 and 30 grains, and HYOSCYAMIN 1–30 grains were given to quiet him. SULPHATE of STRYCHNINE was administered, in gradually increased doses, from 1–60 to 1/3 grain three times daily, hypodermically in the temples. The knee jerk and other reflexes returned. Occasionally he would describe quite accurately some object in the room, but these returns of vision were very transient. His intellect improved materially, as did also his physical condition. About November 1, he had two quite marked convulsions, and we decreased the STRYCHNINE. The patient died late in December of bronchitis and edema of the lungs; a condition not unlike senile bronchitis.

Was this a case of toxic amblyopia [dimness of vision without detectable organic lesion of the eye]? and if so, was it due to QUININE, MORPHINE or WHISKEY? [Amblyopia may also be caused by STRYCHNINE.]

———

Appendix H

Appendix I
Why Teach Materia Medica?

by
W. A. George, M.D.
Member of the Teaching Staff
of the
College of Medical Evangelists, 1912.

In this article the subject of Materia Medica is treated entirely from the standpoint of those who are in every way possible attempting to reduce the use of drugs to a minimum, and not from the standpoint of the physician who depends almost entirely upon drugs in the treatment of disease.

The teaching of this subject may be divided for our purpose according to the following outline:

Materia Medica

1. Toxicology
    A. Signs and tests of poisons
    B. Antidotes
2. Physiological actions
    A. Effects of drugs
    B. Effects of other remedies
3. Therapeutic uses
    A. Necessary
    B. Emergencies
    C. Removal of drugs
4. Dangers
    A. Extreme ideas
    B. Depending on drugs

1. Toxicology.
    A. It is certainly evident to all that every physician and nurse should understand the signs and symptoms of poisoning by various drugs and chemicals used ordinarily as medicine. Physicians should also understand the various tests for poisons which may be taken with suicidal

intent or accidentally. If from this standpoint only we were to teach Materia Medica, we have every reason to urge every medical student to spend enough time to become familiar with this phase of the subject.

B. It is also evident that every physician and nurse should understand the simple antidotes which may be used to relieve those suffering from poisoning. Under the heading of Toxicology we might also consider the importance of understanding the effects of all drugs which are ordinarily given, even though not in lethal doses but which leave their signs and symptoms behind, and unless their effects are understood, one is liable to mistake the effect of the drug for some disease. It is often necessary to examine a patient who is suffering from the influence of drugs more than from any ordinary disease, and in these cases, if the physician does not thoroughly understand the effects of these drugs, he will be led astray and perhaps make a wrong diagnosis.

2. Physiological actions.

A. Effects of drugs. In the study of Materia Medica and Therapeutics many men have spent years in working out the effects of various drugs, and their efforts are surely of great value in aiding the physician in the study of disease and the desired effects which we may wish to secure in the treatment of disease. While in many cases we may simply study the use of the remedy from the standpoint of those who give the drugs and yet not intend to give them ourselves, it is important to know what would be produced by the administration of these drugs so that we may compare their effects with—

B. The effects of other remedies. In our efforts to treat disease without the use of drugs, we should receive great benefit by comparing the effects of drugs with the effects of physiological remedies such as hydrotherapy, massage, exercise, electricity, etc. When we study in Materia Medica the effects of the various classes of drugs, we should then compare these with similar effects produced by simple physiological remedies without the use of poisonous drugs. In this way the student will be led to adopt the simpler method and discard the use of drugs.

3. Therapeutic uses.

A. Necessary. Under the necessary use of drugs may be placed anesthetics, antiseptics, and various useful remedies which may be applied externally both for the protection of injured parts and for the relief of pain. Every physician should study carefully the safest and most effectual means of administering an anesthetic under various conditions.

Appendix J

He should also thoroughly understand the nature of antiseptics and their use both externally and internally as applied to abseses, cavities, etc.

B. Emergencies. There are certainly times when some simple drug given in sufficient quantity to produce a desired result may be administered with less danger and with better results than can be accomplished by the use of other measures. When it becomes necessary in the mind of the physician to resort to a drug, he should do so only after carefully considering the possible results and dangers which may follow either the use of the drug or the attempt to relieve the patient without the drug remedy.

C. Removal of drugs. We frequently have cases coming to us who have been using certain drugs as prescribed by other physicians. There are cases where to remove the drug at once may prove a great injury to the patient, and while these cases may be exceptional, yet it is certainly better to give a few doses of some drug which the patient has been taking before than to run the risk either of serious injury to the patient or possibly of losing the chance to treat the case, as some will not yield to the complete removal at once. Under these conditions a physician is certainly justified in giving a few doses, perhaps reduced in quantity, while he is getting the patient under other forms of treatment.

4. Dangers.

A. Extreme ideas. While we are attempting to treat disease as far as possible without the use of drugs, it would certainly be extreme for anyone to teach that drugs of every form should never be given under any conditions. There are certainly many cases where, as related above, it may be absolutely necessary to resort to the use of some simple drug remedy, and the idea should not be given out by anyone that our physicians never use any drug remedy.

B. Depending on drugs. Perhaps the greatest danger among our physicians is the growing habit of depending upon the use of drugs. While we claim to use drugs for internal purposes to a very limited extent only, there is danger after giving a certain remedy in some case where we feel that we are obliged to do so, that it will be easier to give the same drug to other cases later, and thus the habit is formed of prescribing certain drug remedies quite frequently. This is by all means the greatest danger among our physicians, and the importance of avoiding the use of drugs excepting in extreme cases should be most thoroughly impressed upon our students. The more thorough the understanding of Materia Medica the more carefully it is taught to medical students, and at the same time the dangers of the use of drugs pointed out, the more these students will be prepared to resist the temptation of resorting to drugs.

It should be impressed upon students that "drugs never cure disease," that they "only change the form and location of disease," and while we sometimes resort to certain drugs in an emergency, we do not do so because we think the drugs will especially benefit the patient, but, as in the case of an anesthetic, we know there will be an injury but we have the choice of an injury by the drug or not being able to relieve the patient by necessary surgical work. In other cases we may resort to some remedy as a cathartic or laxative in a surgical case, or an accident case where the patient cannot be moved or where he cannot take food which will bring about the desired results; but even in these cases the student should be taught that the medicine leaves a bad effect and to continue the drug will only prove an injury.

Students and young physicians cannot be impressed too strongly with the dangers of relying upon poisonous drugs for the cure of disease. There are undoubtedly many cases where the physician almost thoughtlessly resorts to some drug which is simple to give and required very little study on his part, yet if he were to study more thoroughly he would be able to prescribe some treatment which would relieve the patient without the use of drugs, and thereby accomplish not only the relief of the patient, leaving no evil effects behind, but also impress upon both nurse and patient as well as the friends and society at large, the value of simple remedies when given under the blessing of God. Undoubtedly careful, prayerful study and depending upon God's blessing in the administration of the God-given remedies of which we have had the privilege of learning would cure many cases where the administration of drugs has not accomplished the desired result and patients have gone away disappointed. Above all, our students should he taught that God's blessing added to our humble efforts when we have done the best we can with simple remedies will always accomplish more than drugs in any form, and while there may be emergencies when we will think it best to prescribe some drug, this should only be done after careful and prayerful consideration of the results to follow and after exhausting all our resources in attempting to relieve the condition by a simpler method.

The Medical Evangelist, January, 1912, 9–12.

Appendix J

As We Go to Press

The following references were located too late to be included in their proper order with the other references. They are, however, included properly in the indexes.

1890—*Manuscript Release No 1033: The Salamanca Vision and the 1890 Diary,* 17.

"We were delayed one day longer than we designed. I had ague in my ear, and head was involved. I suffered much pain. Dared not be on the road. I consulted a dentist. He said the teeth were not the cause of this affliction. Then I took ALCOHOL, sweat, and worked my best to subdue the pain, and the relief came. I am made aware that all this trouble was the result of a severe cold. . . .

"I have been urging my prayer for the Lord to strengthen me, to give my poor heart a rest from pain. I leave my petition at the throne of grace and say, 'Not my will, but Thine, O Lord, be done.' If it be His pleasure to give me grace to work for Him in pain and suffering almost constantly and this is best for me, I say, 'Amen.' I will continue to work until I lay off the armor at the feet of my Redeemer."

1897—*Manuscript Releases,* vol. 20, 280.

"I send you at this time pulverized CHARCOAL. Let him drink the water after it has stood a while to EXTRACT the VIRTUE. This should be cold when used. When used for fomentations over the bowels, the coal should be put into a bag, sewed up, and dipped in hot water. It will serve several times. Have two bags; use one and then the other."

1898—*Manuscript 45,* 1898, 5.

"Long names have been given to the DRUGS that physicians handle, which no human being should consent to use until he has tried simple, natural remedies."

1899—*Selected Messages,* book 2, 299–300.

"We need a hospital so much. On Thursday Sister Sara McEnterfer was called to see if she could do anything for Brother B's little son, who is eighteen months old. For several days he has had a painful swelling on the knee, supposed to be from the bite of some poisonous insect. Pulverized CHARCOAL, mixed with FLAXSEED, was placed upon the swelling, and this poultice gave relief at once. The child had screamed with pain

all night, but when this was applied, he slept. Today she has been to see the little one twice. She opened the swelling in two places, and a large amount of yellow matter and blood was discharged freely. The child was relieved of its great suffering. We thank the Lord that we may become intelligent in using the simple things within our reach to alleviate pain, and successfully remove its cause."
(*The Paulson Collection of Ellen G. White Letters, 15*)

1906—*Loma Linda Messages*, 155.

"Elder Haskell has suffered a great deal from boils. He has taken treatment at the Sanitarium several times, but most of his treatment he has taken in his room in our house. Our home has been his sanitarium. He has been afflicted continuously, and has kept to his bed most of the time. Pulverized CHARCOAL poultices have been used with good results. His wife is a good nurse, and she has taken faithful care of him. He has thought several times that he had overcome the affliction, and that he would recover rapidly, but as soon as he began to stir around, boils would again appear. His countenance looks clear and wholesome for a man of his age."

1910—*Review and Herald*, January 20, 1910—Willie White, son of E. G. White.

"The day following this almost sleepless night was uneventful. The train glided swiftly along through western Utah and Nevada. Shortly before daylight Thursday morning, September 9, when the train had passed the highest altitude, and was just finishing its run through forty miles of tunnels and snowsheds, Miss McEnterfer, whose berth was nearly opposite, and some others near by, heard agonized groans from Mrs. White. When asked what was the matter, she said she must have air, she could not breathe. But her window was open, and the berth was filled with smoky air from the snow-shed.

"Knowing that we were then seven thousand feet above sea-level, and that we had been several hours in this high altitude, we recognized the difficulty as heart failure, and trembled for the outcome. Miss McEnterfer attempted to count her pulse, but found that impossible, as there was only a little quiver instead of a regular beat. This grew more and more faint. She asked her several questions, but there was no answer. Her hearing and her speech had gone. Her limbs were cold, and she seemed powerless.

"The porter brought some HOT WATER. Into this Miss McEnterfer put a little PEPPERMINT, and with much difficulty got Mrs. White to swallow a few spoonfuls. then she vigorously rubbed her hands and arms and feet. After much delay bottles of hot water were secured and placed over her heart and at her feet. In the course of an hour her pulse began to grow stronger, and as we dropped into the lower altitude, her heart action increased. An hour later as we neared Colfax, she had so far recovered as to be able to speak and to hear what we said to her. During the day she was able to take a little liquid food, and at Oakland Pier and Vallejo Junction made the transfers with the aid of the wheelchairs furnished by the railway company. Arriving at St. Helena at 7 P.M., she walked from the train to her carriage, and was soon in her own home, from which she had been absent five months."

1896—*Pamphlet 31, Extracts from Unpublished Testimonies in Regard to Flesh Foods, 4, 5.*

"There is an alarming lethargy shown on the subject of unconscious sensualism. It is customary to eat the flesh of dead animals. This stimulates the lower passions of the human organism. In the preparation of food, the golden rays of light are to be kept shining, teaching those who sit at the table how to live. Physicians are not employed to prescribe a flesh diet for patients, for it is this kind of diet that has made them sick. Seek the Lord. When you find him, you will be meek and lowly of heart. Individually, you will not subsist upon the flesh of dead animals, neither will you put one morsel in the mouth of your children. You will not prescribe flesh, TEA, or COFFEE for your patients, but will give talks in the parlor showing the necessity of a simple diet. You will cut away injurious things from your bill of fare. To have the physicians of our institutions educating, by precept and example, those under their care to use a meat diet, after years of instruction from the Lord, disqualifies them to be superintendents {5} of our health institutes. The Lord does not give light on health reform that it may be disregarded by those who are in positions of influence and authority. The Lord means just what he says, and he is to be honored in what he says. Light is to be given upon these subjects. It is the diet question that needs close investigation, and prescriptions should be made in accordance with health principles."

Spirit of Prophecy References

1896—*Pamphlet 31, Extracts from Unpublished Testimonies in Regard to Flesh Foods,* 6.

"When a limb is broken, physicians recommend their patients not to eat meat, as there will be danger of inflammation setting in. Condiments and spices used in the preparation of food for the table aid in digestion in the same way that TEA, COFFEE, and LIQUOR are supposed to help the laboring man perform his tasks. After the immediate effects are gone, they drop as correspondingly below par as they were elevated above par by these STIMULATING SUBSTANCES. The system is weakened, the blood is contaminated, and inflammation is the sure result."

1900—*A Call To Stand Apart,* 23.

"The pursuit of pleasure and amusement centers in the cities. Many parents who choose a city home for their children, thinking to give them greater advantages, meet with disappointment, and too late repent their terrible mistake. The cities of today are fast becoming like Sodom and Gomorrah. The many holidays encourage idleness. The exciting sports—theatergoing, horse racing, gambling, LIQUOR-DRINKING, and reveling—stimulate every passion to intense activity. The youth are swept away by the popular current. Those who learn to love amusement for its own sake open the door to a flood of temptations. They give themselves up to social gaiety and thoughtless mirth, and their intercourse with pleasure lovers has an INTOXICATING effect upon the mind. They are led on from one form of dissipation to another, until they lose both the desire and the capacity for a life of usefulness. Their religious aspirations are chilled; their spiritual life is darkened. All the nobler faculties of the soul, all that link man with the spiritual world, are debased."

1907—*Last Day Events,* 23.

We know that the Lord is coming very soon. The world is fast becoming as it was in the days of Noah. It is given over to selfish indulgence. Eating and drinking are carried to excess. Men are drinking the POISONOUS LIQUOR that makes them mad.—Letter 308, 1907."

Spirit of Prophecy References

Index

Page numbers with an asterix (*) are not occurrences of Ellen G. White's words or are not attributed to her.

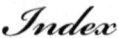

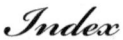

O

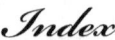

Index

Index of Diseases

Page numbers with an asterix (*) are not occurrences of Ellen G. White's words or are not attributed to her.

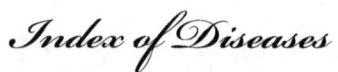

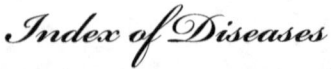

Index of Diseases

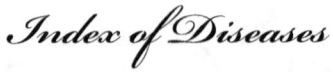

Index of Diseases

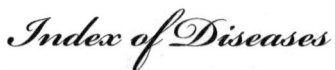

Index of Diseases

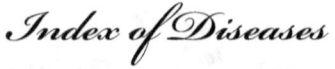

Index of Diseases

thirst, raging 58
throat enfeebled 129
   throat, trouble with 11, 153, 160, 164
tobacco, air poisoned by 61
tongue, paralysis of 104
   thick and swollen 26
tuberculous, see consumption
tumors 29
typhoid fever 99, 121, 122

U

ulcers 14, 29
   dreadful 17
unconsciousness 78, 183*
   from second hand tobacco smoke 61
urine very scanty 208*

V

vision 208*
   vision, loss of 28

vital energies exhausted 32
vital energy 109
vital force, kill the remaining 100
   little 19, 36
vital forces, destroy the 71
   exhausted 29
   wearing away of 83
vitality, decreasing rapidly 23
   destroying their 44
   extinguishing the spark of 66
   physical, is undermined 91
vomiting 79

W

weakness 16, 18, 74
weary, very 19
white blood cells 178*
women, diseases of 159, 163
wrecks, useless 22
wretchedness 17

www.ingramcontent.com/pod-product-compliance
Lightning Source LLC
Chambersburg PA
CBHW060244290526
45789CB00001B/180